Antonio Barquet

Traumatic Hip Dislocation in Childhood

With a Foreword by Roberto Masliah

With 56 Figures

Springer-Verlag
Berlin Heidelberg New York
London Paris Tokyo

Dr. ANTONIO BARQUET
Department of Orthopedics and Traumatology
University of Montevideo
Montevideo - Uruguay

ISBN-13:978-3-642-82894-2 e-ISBN-13:978-3-642-82892-8
DOI: 10.1007/978-3-642-82892-8

Library of Congress Cataloging in Publication Data

Barquet, Antonio, 1947-
Traumatic hip dislocation in childhood.

Bibliography: p.
Includes index.
1. Hip joint - Dislocation. 2. Hip joint - Fractures. 3. Children - Wounds and injuries - Complications and sequelae. I. Title.
[DNLM: 1. Hip Dislocation - complications. 2. Hip Dislocation - in infancy & childhood. 3. Hip Fractures - in infancy & childhood. WE 860 B267t]
RD549.B37 1986 617'.581044 86-31610

Reproduction of the figures: Gustav Dreher GmbH, Stuttgart

2124/3130-543210

To my wife Pilar and
my daughter Carolina

To my Parents

Foreword

Although the number of published papers on traumatic hip dislocation in childhood is large, our actual current knowledge on this injury in this age group is still full of obscure points and unsolved problems. Luxation of the hip of traumatic origin in children is infrequent, and the small number of cases reported by authors and institutions, as well as the usually short follow-up in many cases, are responsible for the many doubts and questions, especially related to complications and outcome following the injury. Consequently the treatment, especially the postreduction management, has not been adequately defined.

Dr. Antonio Barquet has made the great effort to analyze the experience gained from 38 cases in Uruguay and to review more than 500 references related to the subject, covering more than 1400 cases.

He began to study this topic in 1976. It was the subject of his postgraduate monograph in 1979, which was followed by a statistical analysis of the major complication, i. e., avascular necrosis of the proximal femoral extremity, which was presented as his doctoral thesis in 1981. In addition, he has published numerous papers dealing with several aspects of traumatic hip dislocation in children.

The reader will find in this book a personal "mise au point" of this injury in children, based on the author's experience and on everything he has read and considered during all these years. The book describes a series of conclusions and defines many of the above-mentioned obscure points and problems. For instance, the therapeutic protocol established in this book is to be highly recommended, and the analysis and conclusions on complications are outstanding. Undoubtedly, there are still other difficulties whose clarification will become possible with the passing of time, together with further observation and analysis of cases and new facts.

We congratulate Dr. Barquet on this presentation, and we would like to say that this book will not only be an extremely useful source of consultation for all those orthopedic surgeons confronted with a child presenting a traumatic dislocation of the hip, but also a very important basis for all those who wish to go on studying this theme.

ROBERTO MASLIAH

Preface

"Traumatic hip dislocation in childhood is rare.... The follow-up, a significant factor, is usually too brief. Therefore, hip joint behaviour after traumatic hip dislocation in this age group has not been adequately documented in order to provide defined therapeutic principles" [21]. These facts, together with certain essential characteristics of traumatic dislocations of the developing hip, have led to significant controversies about associated lesions, complications and, of course, treatment. This is complicated by another factor: "Seldom does a child suffer traumatic dislocation of the hip. It is virtually impossible for any one physician to study a sufficient number of cases personally.... Our information must depend upon sufficient accumulated material derived from well documented and adequately followed cases" [370]. A further complication is the fact that the information on this injury in children is widely dispersed in the literature and no attempt has been made to collect all these data in a single manuscript.

I have based my study on the experience gained with a significant number of cases treated in my country in the last 30 years, especially with those in which I was fortunate to obtain a long term follow-up. Just as importantly, it is also based on the data that I have collected in a thorough review of the international literature, including written information and the evaluations of cases. This work was essential in order to analyze, evaluate, and think about these questions.

I have tried to present the different aspects of traumatic hip dislocation in childhood which are mentioned in the vast literature, and have put particular emphasis on the special characteristics of this injury in childhood, the controversies and problems mentioned above, and my personal views and thoughts about them.

I am most grateful to N. Castiglioni, R. Masliah, and A. Silveri for encouraging me in my studies on traumatic dislocation of the hip in children. Dr. Masliah also read the manuscript, made helpful suggestions and kindly wrote the foreword. V. Vécsei, from Vienna, discussed several aspects of the subject with me.

I am indebted to all the orthopedic surgeons and institutions, both from my country and from abroad, who have contributed cases. Numerous librarians and institutions were very kind in helping me to obtain the large number of references reviewed. I especially want to thank all of them.

D. Giammarchi performed the statistical analysis of the collected data and discussed findings with me.

I am most grateful to A. Cordero, who produced all follow-up roentgenograms in patients from my country and also many of the photographs illustrating this book.

Several authors, journals, and publishing houses very kindly granted permission to use previously published material and provided me with original copies.

It is a pleasure to acknowledge R. Cepellini, H. Schenone, J. H. Leborgne, F. Leborgne and G. Bossano, for reasons well known to them.

I wish to thank W. Bandi and L. Negri, who encouraged me to write this book and presented my plan and project to Springer-Verlag.

I would like to thank Springer-Verlag for its cooperation and for the presentation of this book.

Montevideo ANTONIO BARQUET

Contents

1 Introduction

1.1 General Considerations and Purpose

Traumatic hip dislocation in childhood (THDC) is defined as a traumatic permanent displacement of a previously normal femoral head out of a previously normal acetabulum in individuals under 16 years of age. Dislocations with predisposing pathological factors, such as congenital, septic, or paralytic, are excluded. Central dislocations are also excluded, as the hip is not truly dislocated; instead, there is a fracture of the acetabulum and the joint is displaced medially with respect to the rest of the pelvis [383, 400]. An age limit of 15 years has been chosen as a dividing line between children and adults, because in the group of individuals up to this age the proximal femoral growth plate is still open [20, 21, 146, 161, 185, 302, 306, 308, 322, 365, 411, 438, 448]. With few exceptions this age limit has been uniformly applied in the literature.

Even though the incidence of THDC has increased in recent decades, this injury continues to be uncommon. However, few rare injuries have been the subject of such a large number of publications in the world literature as THDC. The special condition of the maturing hipjoint leads to certain distinguishing characteristics of THDC, differentiating it from the same lesion in adults, with respect to the severity of the causative trauma, the incidence of associated fractures at the joint, and complications related to the perturbance of growth - in part due to mechanical reasons, but especially to vascular damage with compromise of the capital epiphysis and the growth plate - leading to progressive deformity and sequelae in the future life of these children.

There is another main reason for the large number of papers and excellent reviews on THDC: controversy surrounds several important aspects, especially the factors influencing the incidence of complications and the outcome, and consequently the ideal treatment for this injury in children. Although there is general agreement about the imperious need for early reduction of the luxation, there is wide controversy about the role of closed and surgical procedures in simple dislocations and fracture dislocations (FD), the type of postreduction management of these injuries, and the treatment of complications following dislocation.

Thirty-eight cases of THDC from Uruguay have been collected and reviewed along with more than 1400 cases from the literature. The literature on THDC has also been thoroughly investigated. The results of the analysis of this information has been partially presented in previous publications [20–27, 29, 31].

In the following chapters different aspects of THDC will be considered, and I shall predominantly concentrate on the special characteristics of this injury in children, as well as on the controversial facts mentioned above. In this chapter I will provide a short review of hip development and vascularity.

1.2 Hip Development

Several excellent papers have dealt with this subject in recent years [107, 135, 349, 350, 457, 477]. The description which follows is very brief, and its purpose is only to emphasize certain facts which are applicable to the analysis of THDC, its complications and outcome.

1.2.1 Acetabulum

The development of the acetabulum is chiefly determined by a complex growth plate, i.e., the triradiate cartilage (also called Y-growth plate), which represents the confluence of the three growth plates of the innominate bone, i.e., iliac, public, and ischial (Fig. 1.1). These three sectors are thus integrated in their development, which is centered at the future acetabular socket. These growth plates function physiologically by appositional multiplication of cells. It is interesting to note that there is prolonged interstitial expansion of physis and epiphysis, because the metaphyseal bone does not elaborate a subchondral plate until late in development [350]. Then, continuous growth of the acetabulum, congruous with the development of the femoral head, occurs.

The superior third of the iliac bone, the posterior part of the ischial bone, and the pubic bone represent secondary ossification centers which appear in adolescence. There is also a secondary ossification nucleus for the acetabular rim, i.e., the os acetabuli.

1.2.2 Proximal End of Femur

At birth, the capital epiphysis and the greater trochanter comprise a continuous mass of cartilage (Fig. 1.2a). There is no femoral neck. This chondroepiphysis is separated from the metaphyseal bone by the growth plate (so-called physis, of half-moon nature), with a superior-medial part in front of the femoral head, and a superior-lateral part in front of the greater trochanter. The capsule of the hip joint attaches along the intertrochanteric region anteriorly, posteriorly, and superiorly, but inferiorly just above the lesser trochanter [350].

The growth plate progressively modifies its shape, because there is a significant development of the femoral neck due to a more rapid growth of the medial side of the physis and metaphysis (Fig. 1.2b, c). The separation between the capital epiphysis and the greater trochanter increases. The medial side of the growth plate, i.e., the longitudinal growth plate (LGP), lengthens the neck (Fig. 1.2d). The lateral side of the growth plate, i.e., the trochanteric growth plate (TGP), and the intermediate part between the LGP and the TGP, i.e., the femoral neck isthmus (FNI) - which continues the direction of the TGP - widen the femoral neck (Fig. 1.2d). It should

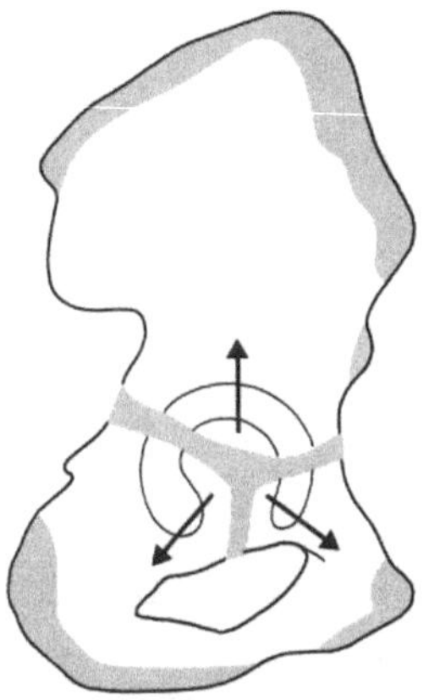

Fig. 1.1. Development of innominate bone. *Shaded areas* represent areas of growth cartilage. Centrifugal ossification - appositional growth - of ilium, ischium, and pubis is centered at the future acetabular socket

be noted that both the TGP and the FNI lengthen significantly more than the LGP, due to the more rapid growth of the medial side of the plate (Fig. 1.2c, d).

The *capital femoral ossific nucleus* appears between 4 and 6 months of age (Fig. 1.2). The growth cartilage at the capital epiphysis functions as a "round" growth center, with the peripheral cells of the columns immediately under the joint cartilage (Fig. 1.2). The capital ossific nucleus, at the center of the capital epiphysis, corresponds to the ossification part of the growth center, which in this part of the proximal femur is initially of a spherical shape. The femoral head enlarges because of appositional multiplication of surface cartilage cells nourished by joint fluid; thus ossification is centrifugal. The capital ossific nucleus progressively enlarges, though more in a transverse direction than vertical, creating a hemispherical shape instead of the original spherical one (Fig. 1.2c, d). This occurs at 4 years of age. From then on, the capital ossific nucleus continues to enlarge in its hemispherical shape, and the cartilaginous mass of the epiphysis becomes progressively filled with bone. At 13-14 years of age the capital epiphysis extends over and around the metaphysis medially, anteriorly, and posteriorly (Fig. 1.2e). However, only the epiphysis is covered by articular cartilage, i.e., the definite femoral head.

The continuous growth of the LGP, TGP, and FNI will lead to development of the femoral neck in length and width. The LGP develops much more medially than laterally, and there is a progressive valgus of the capital epiphysis, the plate tending to be more horizontal (Fig. 1.2c). The more rapid development in the length of the femoral neck than in the growth of the greater trochanter determines that the neck becomes much more intraarticular than the trochanter, and also that the articular surface of the capital epiphysis becomes more proximal than the greater trochanter. The development of the neck also leads to a progressively longer TGP and FNI, and to a narrowing and lengthening of the intraepiphyseal hyaline cartilage, intermediate between capital epiphysis and greater trochanter (Fig. 1.2c, d). The interrelationship between LGP (valgus growth of the neck) and TGP-FNI (varus growth of the neck) (Fig. 1.2d) will determine the definitive position of the proximal end of the femur: from the initial valgus position - inclination angle 145° - of the femoral neck in younger children, there is a progressive diminution of this angle, i.e., inward growth, leading to a definitive position of 130° when the growth plate undergoes fusion. There is also a concomitant variation in the anteversion angle, which reaches

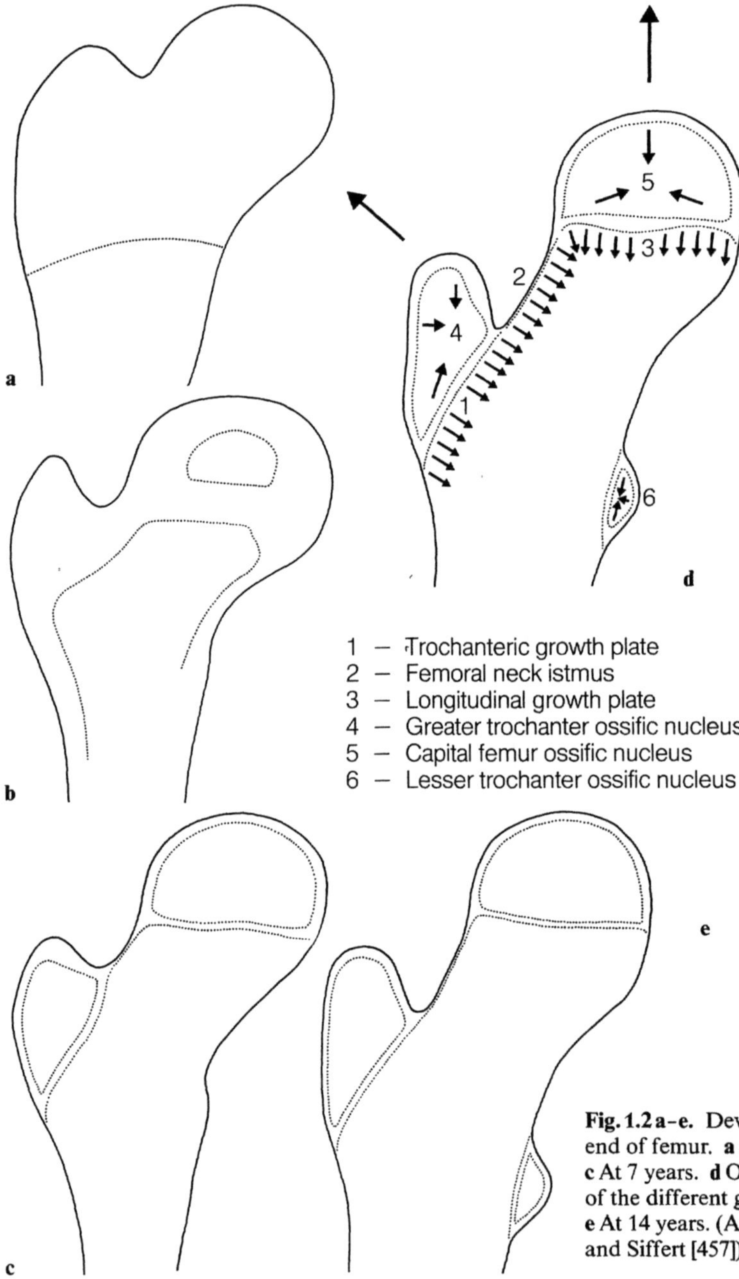

Fig. 1.2 a–e. Development of proximal end of femur. **a** At birth. **b** At 1 year. **c** At 7 years. **d** Ossification "modus" of the different growth centers. **e** At 14 years. (According to Ogden [350] and Siffert [457])

40° at birth, and progressively diminishes to 10° when the growth plates are fused (Fig. 1.2 e).

The *ossific nucleus of the greater trochanter* (Fig. 1.2 c) appears at the cartilaginous mass above the lateral metaphysis at 3 years of age. This secondary nucleus, of the spherical type, is similar to the capital ossific nucleus: it enlarges by appositional growth, i.e., centrifugal ossification (Fig. 1.2 d). The *lesser trochanter* also develops from a secondary ossification center which appears at 8–9 years of age, and grows by centrifugal ossification (Fig. 1.2 d).

As Ogden states, at age 8 or 9 the definite anatomic contours of anteversion, the functionally separated femoral head and trochanter, and the inclination angle are established. Most of the subsequent growth of the proximal end of the femur will consist of interrelated enlargements of the capital epiphysis, trochanter, and neck, as well as remodeling of trabecular patterns [350, 351].

Closure of the growth plate at the proximal end of the femur occurs between the ages of 16 and 17. The LGP is the first to close. Fusion of the TGP begins before closure of the LGP is complete, while the lesser trochanter undergoes fusion concomitant to the greater trochanter.

1.3 Hip Vascularity

The normal vascular distribution in the hip during childhood, especially at the proximal femoral end, plays an important role in the interpretation of complications following THDC – mainly avascular necrosis – as will be shown in Chap. 5. A short description of the most significant aspects of hip vascularity, based on recent investigations by several authors who have performed a *mise au point* of the subject [92, 93, 106, 231, 232, 274, 349, 350, 351], follows (Fig. 1.3).

The arteries of the proximal end of the femur may be described in two groups of quite different significance: (a) the medial and lateral circumflex arteries, which constitute the main vascular supply to this part of the skeleton; and (b) the arteries of the round ligament, which are only a mild complement to the blood supply of the femoral head.

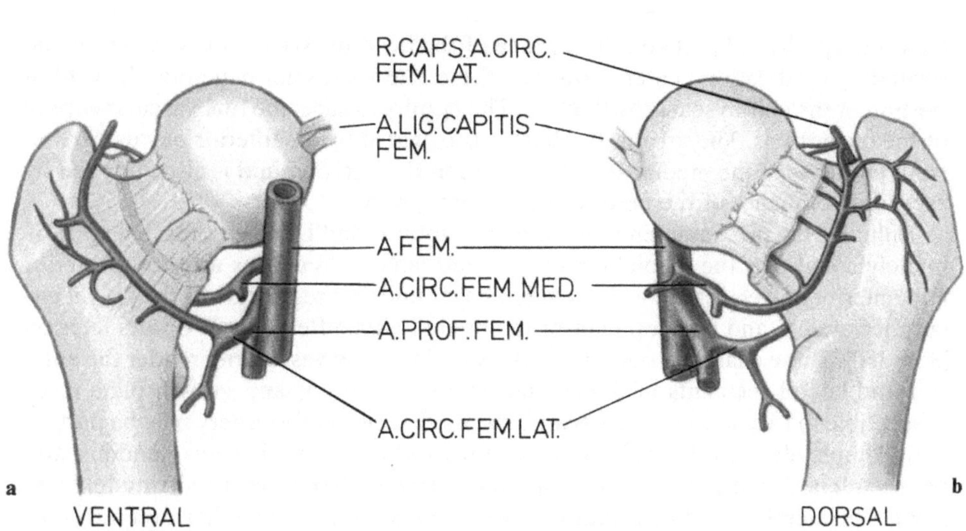

Fig. 1.3 a, b. The blood supply to the proximal end of femur. **a** Ventral, **b** dorsal

The *medial and lateral circumflex arteries* arise either from the femoral or profunda femoris arteries, at the level of the tendinous portion of the iliopsoas muscle. The medial circumflex artery passes between the iliopsoas and pectineus muscles, and then between the medial capsule and the obturator externus muscle. The main branch of this artery goes along the posterior intertrochanteric notch and may cross over to the anterosuperior portion of the intertrochanteric groove, where it anastomoses with the terminal part of the lateral circumflex artery. The lateral circumflex artery, after emerging from the femoral or profunda femoris arteries, crosses the lateral portion of the iliopsoas muscle, to reach the rectus femoris, where it divides into several terminal branches. The transverse branch, the most important, goes over the anterior intertrochanteric notch, and its terminal rami eventually anastomose with the medial circumflex artery at the intertrochanteric notch, as just described.

Therefore, an extracapsular arterial ring results at the base of the neck of the femur, at the level of the capsular attachment of the hip joint, with a posterior half-circumference formed by the medial circumflex artery, completed anteriorly by branches of the lateral circumflex artery. This extracapsular circulation pattern changes very little during growth.

As described by Crock [92] and Chung [106], branches emerge from the extracapsular arterial ring at regular intervals, so-called *ascending cervical arteries,* which traverse the anterior, medial, posterior, and lateral surfaces of the joint capsule close to its insertion into bone. These ascending arteries run upward under the synovial reflection toward the articular cartilage rim, which demarcates the femoral head from the neck, where the arteries anastomose, forming a subsynovial arterial ring. The ascending arteries give rise to metaphyseal and epiphyseal arteries, which provide vascularity to the metaphysis and epiphysis of the upper end of the femur. The *metaphyseal arteries,* disposed in a multitude of very small vessels emerging from the subsynovial ring, are responsible for the blood supply to the metaphysis and the developing femoral neck, both of which are well irrigated. The *epiphyseal arteries* cross the epiphyseal plate on the surface of the head-neck junction and supply the secondary ossification center. However, these arteries do not penetrate the central portion of the epiphyseal growth plate. The epiphysis lacks the fine vascular supply of the metaphysis. The greater trochanter is irrigated by an anterior plexus derived from branches of the medial and lateral circumflex arteries, and is also supplied by ascending branches of the perforating arterial system.

Initially, the proximal femoral chondroepiphysis and LGP are supplied approximately equally by the medial circumflex and lateral circumflex arteries (posterior and anterior halves, respectively). Ogden has found that regression of the lateral circumflex system and development of the medial circumflex system occurs later on [349, 350]. These changing patterns of proximal femoral vascularity render the anterior and lateral segments of the capital femoral epiphysis and growth plate more susceptible to vascular injuries because the medial circumflex artery may be partially or completely occluded at its initial extracapsular course - between tendons, and between tendons and bone - in positional extremes, like those occurring in THD [349]. The lateral ascending arteries, mostly dependent on the medial circumflex artery, supply most of the vascularity to the femoral head and neck. This is a single-stem artery which crosses the capsule at the posterior trochanteric fossa; therefore, injuries to this artery may cause significant damage to the proximal end of the femur, and this may also occur in THDC.

As previously stated, the arteries of the round ligament only supplement the blood supply to the perifoveal area of the femoral head, thus being of no clinical significance.

As shown by Chung [106], veins parallel arteries at the proximal end of the femur.

The vascular supply to the acetabulum deserves no deep analysis. This bone is fully irrigated by multiple arterial branches derived from the obturator, ischial, and gluteal arteries. These arterial branches are paralleled by veins.

2 Etiopathogenesis

2.1 Incidence

2.1.1 General Considerations

Although the incidence of THDC has increased in recent decades, mostly related to the escalation in motor vehicle accidents, this injury continues to be uncommon.

Several examples confirm this statement. Table 2.1 shows most of the large series of THDC previously published, and illustrates that even in the larger institutions the number of collected cases is relatively significant only when those children admitted over two or three decades are reviewed together. Except for these series and a few others, each collected from several institutions [172, 185, 370], the literature contains for the most part single case reports, and rarely presentations of short series of cases usually ranging from two or three observations to six, seven or eight.

There are several major reviews of the literature on THDC (see Table 2.2). These reviews have recorded several hundred previously published cases. However, there is superimposition of cases and of series of cases in most reviews, while other observations are not included.

After a thorough review of the world literature, I was able to collect 1404 cases published between 1823 and 1984. To these observations I have added 38 cases collected in Uruguay, some provided by colleagues and institutions, and some personal (30 of these 38 cases have already been published). The pertinent data relative to authors and year of publication of these 1442 cases of THDC - which I have designated as the World Series (WS), a series that will be very useful in numerous sections of this book - is presented in Table 2.3.

2.1.2 Incidence of THDC Relative to THDA

THD is significantly less common in children than in adults: the incidence of THDC is between 4% and 10% of all THD [98, 146, 266, 304, 376, 381]. The reasons why THDC so infrequently occurs appear to be as follows. Children are less exposed to violence and to those traumas which generally cause THD than adults [45, 253, 259, 309, 324, 329, 356, 501]. The ratio of resistance of the capsuloligamentous structures of the joint to that of the bone is greater in children than in adults [68, 186, 324, 405]. The small surface of the fulcrum site where the femoral neck impinges on the acetabular rim makes leverage movement very difficult and inefficient in children, thus diminishing the chances of dislocation of the femoral head from the ace-

Table 2.1. Several large series of cases of THDC published in the literature, illustrating number of cases and period of admittance to institutions

Year	Author	No. of cases	Institution	Period of admittance
1956	Picchio	8	Istituto Ortopedico Rizzoli, Bologna	1901-1956
1958	Jonasch	2	Unfallkrankenhaus Wien	1926-1956
1959	Morton	7	Vancouver General Hospital	1936-1958
1962	Altav	14	Orthopaedic University Clinic, Istambul	1951-1961
1962	Ulloa	10	Hospital Ortopédico Universitario, Concepción	1947-1961
1968	Rigault et al.	12	Hospital des Enfants Malades, Paris	1954-1966
1973	Schlonsky et al.	17	Children's Hospital, Columbus	1950-1971
1974	Robertson et al.	24	Mayo Clinic, Rochester	1938-1971
1975	Chotigavanichaya	17	Siriraj Hospital, Bangkok	1966-1972
1976	Obel et al.	8	Klinika Chirurgii Dzieciecej, Lublin	1965-1975
1976	Macfarlane et al.	23	Middlemore Hospital, Auckland	1949-1972
1977	Kanan et al.	30	Hospital das Clinicas, Sao Paolo	1953-1971
1979	Barquet	20	Instituto y Cátedra Universitaria de Ortopedia y Traumatología, Montevideo	1941-1978
1979	Klasen	10	Groningen University Hospital	1945-1968
1980	Epstein	74	Los Angeles County-University Southern California Medical Center	1928-1976
1981	Canale	44	Campbell Clinic, Memphis	1947-1976
1981	Offierski	33	Hospital for Sick Children, Toronto	1960-1977
1983	Petrini et al.	14	Istituto Ortopedico Toscano, Firenze	1942-1981

tabulum [74, 356, 424]. All these characteristics of the child's hip joint modify as the child grows, approaching the mature condition, thus acquiring the properties of the adult joint and consequently a higher risk and incidence of this injury.

2.1.3 Incidence of THD Relative to Traumatic Separation of the Proximal Femoral Epiphysis and to Femoral Neck Fractures in Children

The correlative incidence of these injuries of the proximal femur in children is a matter of controversy [55, 70, 73, 163, 300, 329, 334, 406, 423, 424]. However, the data at hand seem to confirm a minor incidence of THD compared with femoral neck fracture [20, 73, 163, 329, 334, 423], as well as a significantly lower incidence of traumatic separations than THD [20, 55, 163].

Table 2.2. Major reviews of the literature, collecting previously published cases of THDC

Year	Author	Reference	No. of cases collected	No. of cases reported
1913	Boehnke, E.	50	30	1
1916	Roello, G.	424	35	1
1920	Martel, F.	306	12	1
1921	Doelle, O.	124	37	2
1921	Princeteau, A.[a]	399	15	1
1922	Maffei, F.	300	46	3
1924	Choyce, C.	105	53	6
1924	Maitrejean, M.	302	39	4
1927	Giraud, D.	184	107	2
1954	Mason, M.[b]	309	88	1
1955	Jensen, H.	242	111	1
1956	Fineschi, G.	161	137	7
1958	Barcat, J. et al.	19	209	1
1959	Morton, K.[c]	326	129	7
1962	Ulloa, I.	494	262	10
1965	Bonvallet, J.	55	359	1
1966	Wilson, D.[d]	519	89	4
1967	De Guidi, G. et al.	113	200	3
1968	Donaldson, W. et al.	370	274	49
1974	Brug, E. et al.[e]	58	421	4
1974	Sarungi, P.	438	255	1
1976	Pagano, G. et al.	361	509	2
1979	Barquet, A.	21	500	26
1982	Barquet, A.[f]	28	113	2
1982	Malkawi, H.	304	440	1
1982	Sterling, R. et al.	471	472	20

[a] Obturator dislocations.
[b] Reported cases since 1922, i.e., since Maffei's report.
[c] English literature.
[d] Collected in the 43 years prior to 1966.
[e] Cases published between 1957 (since Fineschi's review) and 1971.
[f] Anterior dislocations.

These findings contradict the previous opinion that the presence of the growth plate, as a locus minoris resistentiae, means that a violent trauma would cause a traumatic separation of the capital epiphysis more frequently than a THDC [19, 111, 113, 186, 306, 329]. This argument has been used by some authors to explain the low incidence of THDC. As a result of the present review, I conclude that this argument is not valid at all.

2.2 Age

There is general agreement nowadays that children of any age may suffer a THD. However, there have been controversial findings and statements concerning the incidence of the injury in the different childhood age groups [45, 98, 104, 146, 162,

Table 2.3. Pertinent data from 1442 collected cases of THDC (The World Series)

Year of publication	Author	No. of cases	Year of publication	Author	No. of cases	Year of publication	Author	No. of cases	Year of publication	Author	No. of cases
1823	Cooper	15	1891	Kummer	1	1911	Curtillet et al.	1	1928	Nathan	1
1833	Bloxham	1	1891	Liber	1	1911	Dollinger	1	1931	Nicolaysen	1
1836	Vetu	1	1891	Ollier	1	1911	Froelich	1	1932	Elmslie	1
1838	Eteve	1	1893	Gerster	1	1912	Roederer	2	1932	Glynn	2
1847	Ormerod	1	1893	Helferich	2	1913	Boehnke	1	1932	Pouzet	2
1852	Wood	1	1893	Kuster	1	1913	Roux	4	1933	Sternberg	1
1855	Dupuis	1	1893	Mikulicz	1	1914	Rischbieth	1	1934	Goetz	1
1855	Malgaigne	1	1893	Volkmann	1	1916	Platt et al.	1	1934	Meng	2
1855	Markoe	1	1895	Burci	1	1916	Roello	1	1934	Phemister	1
1861	Sedillot	2	1895	Spencer	1	1919	Elmslie	1	1935	Mauck et al.	1
1864	Cooke	1	1896	Clark	1	1919	Froelich	1	1936	Blumensaat	1
1866	Delagarde	1	1896	Dixson	1	1920	Guersant	2	1936	Maia	2
1868	Powdrell	1	1896	Drehmann	1	1920	Higgins	1	1937	Cuche	4
1869	Bryant	1	1896	Mouczy	1	1920	Sundt	2	1937	Charry	1
1874	Bartels	2	1897	Rosenberg	1	1921	Doelle	2	1937	Haines	1
1877	Doutrelepont	1	1898	Bell	1	1921	Pietrzikowski	1	1937	Piqué et al.	1
1877	Lawrence	1	1898	Endlich	1	1921	Princeteau	1	1938	Coimbra	6
1878	Bigelow	1	1900	Bajardi	1	1922	Campbell	1	1938	Funsten et al.	3
1878	Post	1	1900	Kaufmann	1	1922	Maffei	3	1938	Goldenberg	1
1878	Williams	1	1900	Perrando	1	1922	Rehbein	1	1938	Michel	1
1884	Hamilton	1	1901	Kirmisson	1	1922	Roello	2	1938	Paltrinieri	1
1884	Jones	1	1901	MacEwen	1	1922	Steinke	1	1938	Pfab	3
1884	Warren	1	1902	Borchard	1	1923	Bassetta	1	1939	Birch-	1
1885	Riedel	1	1902	Tuchten	2	1923	Fairbank	1		Hirschfeld	
1886	Berendes	4	1903	Haedke	1	1923	Murphy	1	1939	Kleinberg	1
1887	Pfeiffer	1	1903	Jalaquier	1	1923	Watkins	1	1939	Mutschler	1
1887	Smith	1	1904	Seiderer	1	1924	Choyce	6	1940	Kroll	1
1888	Catoir	1	1907	Froelich	1	1924	Drevermann	1	1940	Watson-Jones	1
1889	Douglas	1	1907	Karehnke	1	1924	Harris	1	1941	Banks	1
1889	Farrant	1	1907	Truchet	1	1924	Maitrejean	4	1941	Caamaño	4
1889	Kammerer	1	1908	Martel	1	1924	Wilson	1	1942	Blanco	1
1889	Klee	2	1908	Peschties	1	1925	Erlacher	1	1942	Bohler	1
1889	Michelmore	1	1908	Streissler	1	1927	Giraud	2	1945	Quist-Hanssen	3
1889	Schomann	1	1910	Mouchet et al.	2	1927	Williams	1	1946	Elizalde	2
1890	Denetieres	1	1910	Weil	2	1928	Clarke	1	1947	Quist-Hanssen	1

Table 2.3. (continued)

Year of publication	Author	No. of cases	Year of publication	Author	No. of cases	Year of publication	Author	No. of cases	Year of publication	Author	No. of cases
1947	Schiele	1	1957	Bohler	6	1962	Jonasch	2	1967	Sankarankutty	1
1947	Urist	2	1957	Grob	2	1962	Oprandi et al.	1	1967	Scialpi et al.	1
1948	Cofre-Cerda	4	1957	Grobelski	7	1962	Ruffoni	1	1968	Arancio et al.	3
1949	Cauchoix et al.	1	1957	Gui	2	1962	Russe	3	1968	Bergoin et al.	1
1950	Calderon	1	1957	Hamada	2	1962	Ulloa	10	1968	Bonnemaison et al.	1
1950	Lezama	2	1958	Barcat et al.	1	1962	Vrbecky	1	1968	Chapchal	1
1950	Niloff et al.	1	1958	Chigot	1	1963	Vuyfjes	1	1968	Chavatte	9
1950	Ottolenghi	1	1958	Economu et al.	2	1963	Koszla	7	1968	Jungbluth et al.	3
1951	Paus	19	1958	Fevre	1	1963	Liuboshits	3	1968	Lehtonen	12
1951	Trillat et al.	1	1958	Jantzen	1	1963	Ricci et al.	3	1968	Ostapowicz	1
1951	Zarotti	5	1958	Jonasch	2	1964	Aufranc et al.	1	1968	Donaldson et al.	49
1952	Bairov	1	1958	Judet	1	1964	Grigovich	1	1968	Rigault et al.	12
1952	Kucerova	1	1958	Litton et al.	1	1964	Hohmann	1	1969	Body	1
1953	Brunner	1	1958	Rampoldi et al.	1	1964	Liuboshits et al.	1	1969	De Paoli et al.	2
1953	Ghormley et al.	1	1958	Tailhefer	1	1964	Liuboshits et al.	78	1969	Hensley et al.	1
1953	Mackay	1	1960	Carpi	1	1964	Masse et al.	1	1969	Hipp	9
1953	Mau	1	1960	Doljnitzkij	2	1964	Mossakowska	1	1969	Hunter	3
1953	Zarotti et al.	2	1960	Gogler	1	1964	Pizziolo	1	1969	Lesourd	1
1954	Mason	1	1960	Seewald	9	1965	Bonvallet	1	1969	Matsubara	2
1954	Stewart et al.	7	1961	Davalli	2	1965	Dialer	1	1969	Miglietta	1
1955	Ayrolo	1	1961	Freeman	7	1965	Fernández	1	1969	Oprandi	2
1955	Barbieri	1	1961	Glass et al.	47	1965	Motta	2	1969	Spissak et al.	3
1955	Blount	1	1961	Gouin	2	1966	Fries	2	1969	Townsend et al.	1
1955	Giglio	1	1961	Haliburton et al.	1	1966	Giglio et al.	1	1970	Benecke	1
1955	Jensen	1	1961	Piggot	9	1966	Perry	1	1970	Bernhang	1
1955	Loray	1	1961	Schonbauer	1	1966	Wilson	4	1970	Fina et al.	3
1955	Perruelo	1	1961	Titze	6	1967	Byram et al.	6	1970	Gupta et al.	32
1955	Ruiz	1	1961	Tronzo	1	1967	Campailla	3	1970	Nelson	1
1955	Scholder	2	1961	Wadsworth	1	1967	Chigot et al.	7	1970	Vena et al.	2
1955	Slullitel	1	1962	Altav	14	1967	De Guidi et al.	3	1971	Boitzy	1
1955	Stringa	1	1962	Brav	3	1967	Helal et al.	2	1971	Fordyce	1
1956	Andreini	1	1962	Doljnitzkij	1	1967	Milazzo et al.	2	1971	Lam	1
1956	Fineschi	7	1962	Flach et al.	8	1967	Sanguinetti	1	1971	Pizio	2
1956	Picchio	7	1962	Funk	40						
1956	Pouliquen	1									

Table 2.3. (continued)

Year of publication	Author	No. of cases	Year of publication	Author	No. of cases	Year of publication	Author	No. of cases	Year of publication	Author	No. of cases
1971	Pizio	1	1974	Rowe	1	1978	Schoenecker et al.	1	1981	Barquet	1
1972	Gula	1	1974	Sarungi	1	1978	Soares	19	1981	Canale	36
1972	Klems	1	1974	Schwartz et al.	1	1979	Abad	4	1981	Hollingdale	1
1972	Lovell	8	1975	Chotigavanichaya	17	1979	Barquet	26	1981	Offierski	33
1972	Oelrich et al.	2	1975	Kuner	1	1979	Beck	2	1982	Abad et al.	1
1972	Simmons et al.	1	1975	M'Bamali	1	1979	Canale et al.	3	1982	Barquet	2
1973	Gaul	1	1975	Rao et al.	1	1979	Cataldi	1	1982	Klein et al.	1
1973	Hennicke	1	1975	Salina et al.	1	1979	Ciliani	5	1982	Klemm	2
1973	Laskowski et al.	8	1976	Duahime et al.	12	1979	Guillaume	5	1982	Malkawi	1
1973	Pearson et al.	20	1976	Hammelbo	1	1979	Jansen et al.	2	1982	Sterling et al.	20
1973	Prat et al.	3	1976	Labaziewicz	1	1979	Klasen	10	1983	Ekstrand et al.	1
1973	Schlonsky et al.	17	1976	Macfarlane et al.	24	1979	Lavianos	13	1983	Fiddian et al.	2
1974	Amihood	2	1976	Nerubay	1	1979	Pannike	1	1983	Garvan	1
1974	Bijlsma	2	1976	Obel et al.	8	1979	Sandor et al.	1	1983	Petrini et al.	14
1974	Brug et al.	4	1976	Pagano et al.	2	1979	Weigand et al.	7	1983	Rosa	1
1974	Coleman	1	1977	Canale et al.	5	1980	Barquet	1	1983	Seringe et al.	1
1974	Furtak	1	1977	Gypta et al.	1	1980	Bunnell et al.	1	1983	Shina et al.	52
1974	Hovelius	2	1977	Johner et al.	2	1980	Epstein	74	1984	Barquet et al.	2
1974	Lugger	1	1977	Rogala et al.	1	1980	Fernandez	7	1984	Barquet	6
1974	Muller	1	1978	Coello et al.	6	1980	Germaneau et al.	10	1984	Collado et al.	1
1974	Proctor	8	1978	Fardon	1	1980	Gupta et al.	18	1984	Floyd	1
1974	Rang	2	1978	Hidalgos	2	1980	Hidalgos	16	1984	Rees et al.	2
1974	Robertson et al.	20	1978	Kanan et al.	30	1980	Mass et al.	7	1984	Ritter et al.	9

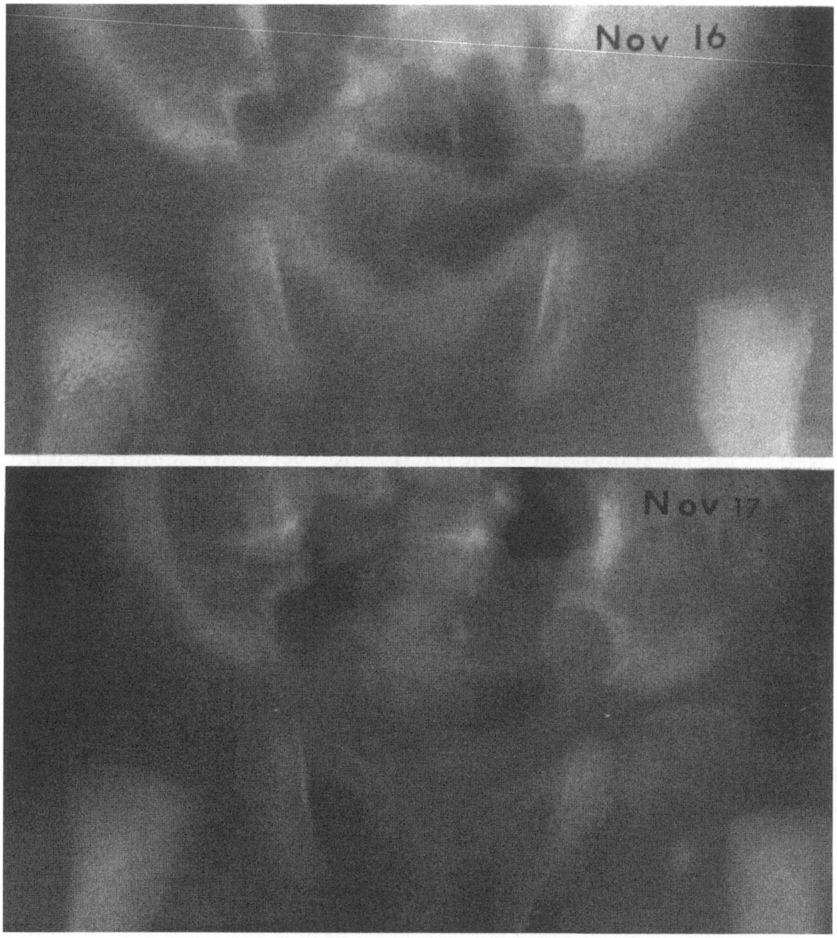

a

b

Fig. 2.1 a, b. Obstetric separation of the proximal femoral epiphysis as a result of a difficult delivery. **a** Characteristic radiographical appearance of this injury, with displacement of the femur resembling a hip dislocation. **b** Arthrogram shows no evidence of dislocation: cartilaginous femoral head is well seated in the normal acetabular socket, but there is epiphyseal separation. (Reprinted from Azouz [13 a])

163, 172, 184, 185, 253, 292, 298, 322, 326, 348, 366, 420, 441, 448]. The analysis of large statistical reviews in the literature resulted in uniform data. Donaldson et al. found, in a combined series of 165 children, that the ages at the time of dislocation were equally distributed within the three 5-year periods between 0 and 15 [370]. Brug and Ziegelmuller reviewed 471 cases and found a similar distribution in these age groups, with a mild predominance in the 6- to 10-year period [58]. The analysis of the WS showed results similar to those of Brug and Ziegelmuller.

Several papers dealing with so-called obstetric THD, including 13 cases reported as such, have been reviewed [3, 174, 195, 267, 298, 336, 369, 391, 394, 413, 475, 505], the dislocation being related to difficult delivery. However, careful evaluation of the available radiographical documentation showed that the obstetric dislocations of the hip appear to be true separations or fracture separations through the physeal region of the proximal femur, as noted by several authors [13a, 53, 111, 237a, 351, 352, 359]. The separation - a Salter type-I epiphyseal cartilage injury, in most instances - occurs at the physis, and the roentgenogram shows a displacement of the femur, resembling a hip dislocation (Fig. 2.1 a). However, an arthrogram confirms the diagnosis of this obstetric fracture as an "apparent dislocation" [13a] (Fig. 2.1 b). In addition, after 1 or 2 weeks a periostic callus appears, which is a further definite diagnostic sign.

2.3 Sex

The ratio between boys and girls, as found in the WS, is 2.5:1, which is similar to previous findings of Morton [326] and Brug and Ziegelmuller [58]. While reviewing the WS from the standpoint of the interrelation between sex and age, it became apparent that, although in the period between 0 and 5 years of age both sexes showed a similar incidence of THD (1:1 ratio) in the subsequent 5-year periods THD significantly and progressively predominated in boys: in the 6- to 10-year period at a 3 to 1 rate, and in the 11- to 15-year period at a rate of 4 to 1.

2.4 Side

There is general agreement about an equal distribution of right and left hip dislocations, and this fact needs no explanation. Bilateral THDC (Fig. 2.2) is exceedingly uncommon. The WS includes only 13 bilateral dislocations [39, 61, 103, 131, 137,

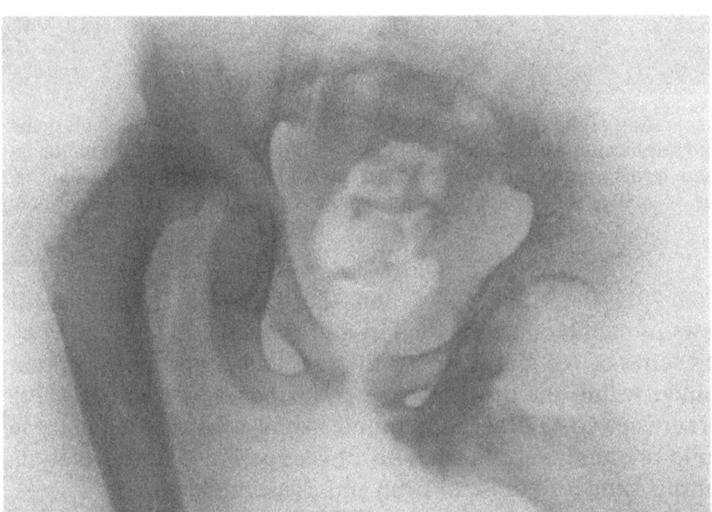

Fig. 2.2. Bilateral traumatic hip dislocation in a 12-year-old child, posterior at the right side, anterior at the left side, with associated avulsion of the greater trochanter. (Reprinted from Economu [137])

146, 277, 291, 320, 378, 393, 420, 522]. The incidence of this "spectacular" injury would thus approach 1% in children, and similar estimates of its incidence in adults have been presented [57, 146].

2.5 Mechanism of Injury

The general conception is that the pathogenic mechanism of THD is similar in children and in adults. Under the influence of a traumatic force, the normal maximal excursion of the joint is surpassed, with capsular laceration and displacement of the femoral head out of the acetabular socket [14, 424, 448].

In general, THD is caused by leverage action, and the different displacement between posterior and anterior dislocations is caused largely by a difference in the anatomic part used as a fulcrum when the dislocation occurs [169, 381, 411, 412, 448, 467], i.e., the anterior acetabular rim in posterior dislocations, and the posterior acetabular rim in anterior dislocations. The usual mechanism acts when the thigh is in adduction-intrarotation (posterior dislocations) or in abduction-extrarotation (anterior dislocations), and an indirect force, longitudinal with respect to the femoral axis, is applied to the hip joint. This axial force is applied either from below, on the knee or the foot, for example when the patient sits in an automobile during a collision or when he falls from a height; or less frequently from above, by heavy weights falling on the torso at the posterior aspect of the pelvis. The altitudinal displacement of the femoral head depends on the position of flexion or extension of the hip joint at the time of injury. When the hip is flexed, the dislocation will be of the low variety: ischial if posterior, and obturator if anterior. When flexion is very mild or when the hip is extended, dislocation will be of the high variety: iliac if posterior, and pubic if anterior. Though infrequently, the force may also be a direct blow to the posterior aspect of the abducted and externally rotated thigh, leading to an anterior dislocation.

In pubic dislocations the mechanism of injury would usually seem to be violent extension or even hyperextension added to abduction-extrarotation of the hip joint, with the femoral head being displaced anteriorly [122].

The mechanism of inferior dislocation, also called luxatio erecta, is an injury forcing the joint into extreme flexion, together with further trauma received on the knee or on the back of the pelvis, but displacing the femur in a caudal direction. Therefore, the femoral head is dislocated below the acetabulum [2].

These previous facts are concerned with so-called regular dislocations, i.e., those in which the Y-ligament is not torn, thus keeping control of the displacement of the femoral head. Irregular dislocations, with the Y-ligament torn, are typical in that the displacement of the femoral head is uncontrolled, and although the general characteristics of posterior and anterior dislocations are maintained, the head comes to lie in atypical positions.

Bilateral dislocations result from analogous mechanisms. However, for a bilateral dislocation to occur, the forces must be distributed between both hips in such a way that they simultaneously deliver sufficient energy to each joint so as to be able to dislocate it.

2.6 Severity of Injury

THDA are uniformly caused by severe injuries. In contrast, a moderate, mild, or even trivial trauma may determine a THD in a child [12, 21, 63, 103, 161, 230, 281, 351, 366, 376, 406, 413, 438, 441]. The severity of the causative trauma of hip dislocation in children is related, in general, to the age of the patient: with increasing age, the trauma tends to be more severe [20, 21, 155, 348, 351, 366, 370, 441]. A review of the WS clearly demonstrates this relationship.

THD in younger children frequently - in fact, in more than 40% of the cases - follows a mild or trivial trauma, i. e., an injury caused by tripping, "doing the splits", falling from the same level, falling out of bed, being pushed by another child, etc. The possibility of easy dislocation of the hip joint in children, mostly occurring in the younger group, is a special characteristic of THDC [12, 21, 63, 101, 103, 107, 146, 163, 185, 222, 230, 281, 351, 366, 391, 407, 411, 420, 438, 441]. These easy dislocations of the hip in younger children occur because of the anatomic properties of the joint in this age group [20, 113, 391, 411, 412, 420]. The hip is less stable in younger children, owing to the pliability of excessive cartilage [113, 351, 385, 391, 412, 420], to the greater elasticity of the capsule and ligaments of the joint [113, 253, 361, 391, 412], and also to a lesser congruity of the joint [179 a, 253, 404, 412]. Concerning the latter, the femoral neck inclination and anteversion in these younger children are very different from those in older children and adults, and the acetabular socket does not display its regularly rounded shape, pertinent depth, and orientation [113, 179 a, 306, 412]. Ralis and McKibbin dissected and measured 44 developing human hip joints and found that this joint is relatively most stable in the embryo, least stable in the perinatal period, and that the stability gradually increases throughout childhood until adult age is reached [404]. A greater muscular laxity in young children has also been mentioned as other factor favoring easy dislocation [257, 361].

In older children, the causative injury of the hip dislocation is more severe. These children usually have their dislocations as a result of high energy or heavy impacts, such as automobile - including so-called dashboard dislocations [174] - or motorcycle accidents, pedestrians being struck by motor vehicles, bicycle accidents, heavy objects falling over the child's back, collapse of buildings, etc. These injuries occur in athletic or sport activities as well, such as football or rugby games, falls from trees or horses, etc.

3 Pathoanatomical Classifications

3.1 By Dislocation

While defining THD, one of the basic criteria is the position of the displaced femoral head with respect to the inhabited acetabulum, i.e., a topographical criterium, and this is identical for adults and children. Allis' classification will be used here. A line drawn from the anterosuperior spine of the ilium through the center of the acetabulum to the ischial tuberosity divides dislocations of the hip into two main groups (Fig. 3.1): when the femoral head is displaced posteriorly to this line, it is designated *posterior;* when the head is in front of this line, it is called *anterior.*

The altitudinal displacement of the femoral head determines the subvariety of posterior and anterior dislocations, namely *high* and *low* posterior and anterior dislocations. Haudidier has added a horizontal line to the schematic criteria for classifying varieties of hip dislocation [215]. She draws a line from the greater sciatic notch through the center of the acetabulum to the upper part of the obturator foramen/ those dislocations with the femoral head lying over this line are high dislocations – iliac when posterior, and pubic when anterior – while those with the femoral head under this line are low dislocations – ischiatic when posterior, and obturator when anterior (Fig. 3.1). An *inferior* variety, also called infracotyloid dislocation or luxatio erecta (Fig. 3.2), will be added.

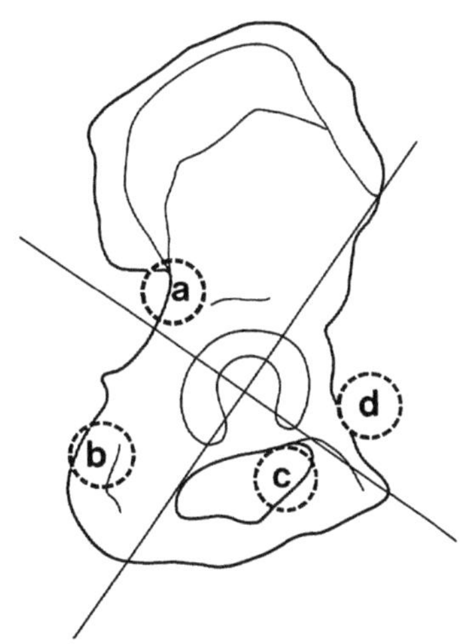

Fig. 3.1. Main varieties of regular traumatic hip dislocation: *a* iliac, *b* ischiatic, *c* obturator, and *d* pubic

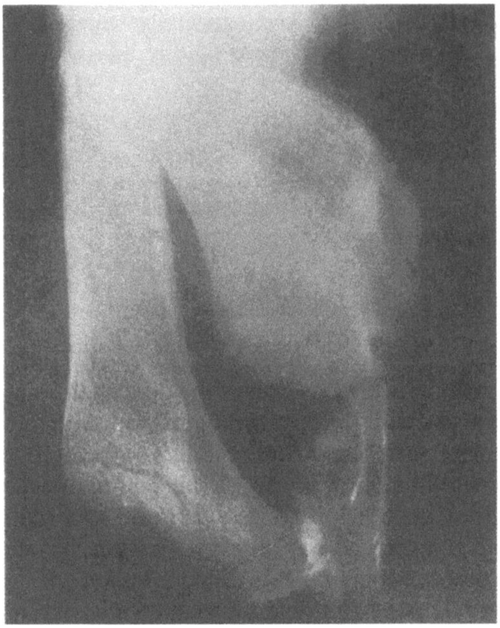

Fig. 3.2. Infracotyloid dislocation (also called luxatio erecta) of the right hip in a 10-year-old boy (From Abad and Barquet [2])

Most dislocations in children are regular, comprised of the iliac and ischiatic posterior varieties, pubic and obturator anterior varieties, and inferior dislocations. In these instances, the Y-ligament is, as already mentioned, intact and the position of the dislocated femoral head is stereotypic with respect to the acetabulum.

Few hip dislocations in this age group involve a random displacement of the head in any direction due to the loss of all restriction of movement, the result of extreme violence and severe rupturing of the ligaments (especially the Y-ligament) and capsule; these are so-called irregular dislocations.

3.1.1 Posterior Dislocations

In posterior dislocations the joint capsule is torn posteriorly by the femoral head, which is displaced in that direction while the femur is in a position of adduction and internal rotation.

Iliac dislocations are high regular posterior dislocations. After moving over the posterior acetabular rim, or fracturing the posterior acetabular rim or wall, the femoral head lies posterosuperiorly along the lateral aspect of the ilium (Fig. 3.3 and 3.4). The limb is in an attitude of adduction, internal rotation, and extension or mild flexion.

High irregular posterior dislocation of the hip is mainly represented by the so-called Monteggia's iliac dislocation or *everted posterior* dislocation. It differs from the usual posterior dislocation because, though the femoral head has been driven posteriorly to the Allis line, the femur is in an attitude of external rotation.

Fig. 3.3. **a** Iliac dislocation of the right hip in an 8-year-old boy following a traffic accident. Closed reduction was achieved within 6 h and skin traction applied for 3 weeks. **b** Twelve years after the injury, there is normal morphology of the hip joint and full, painfree range of motion and unrestricted activities

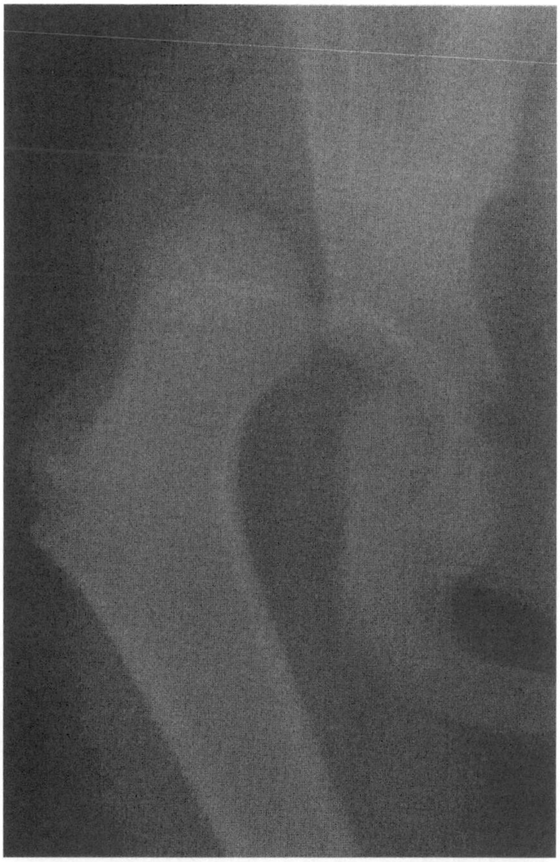

a

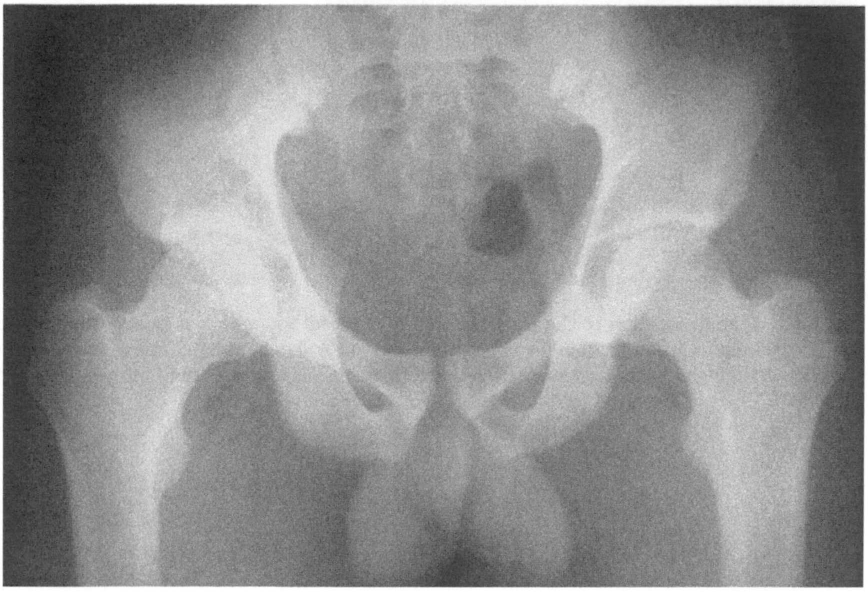

b

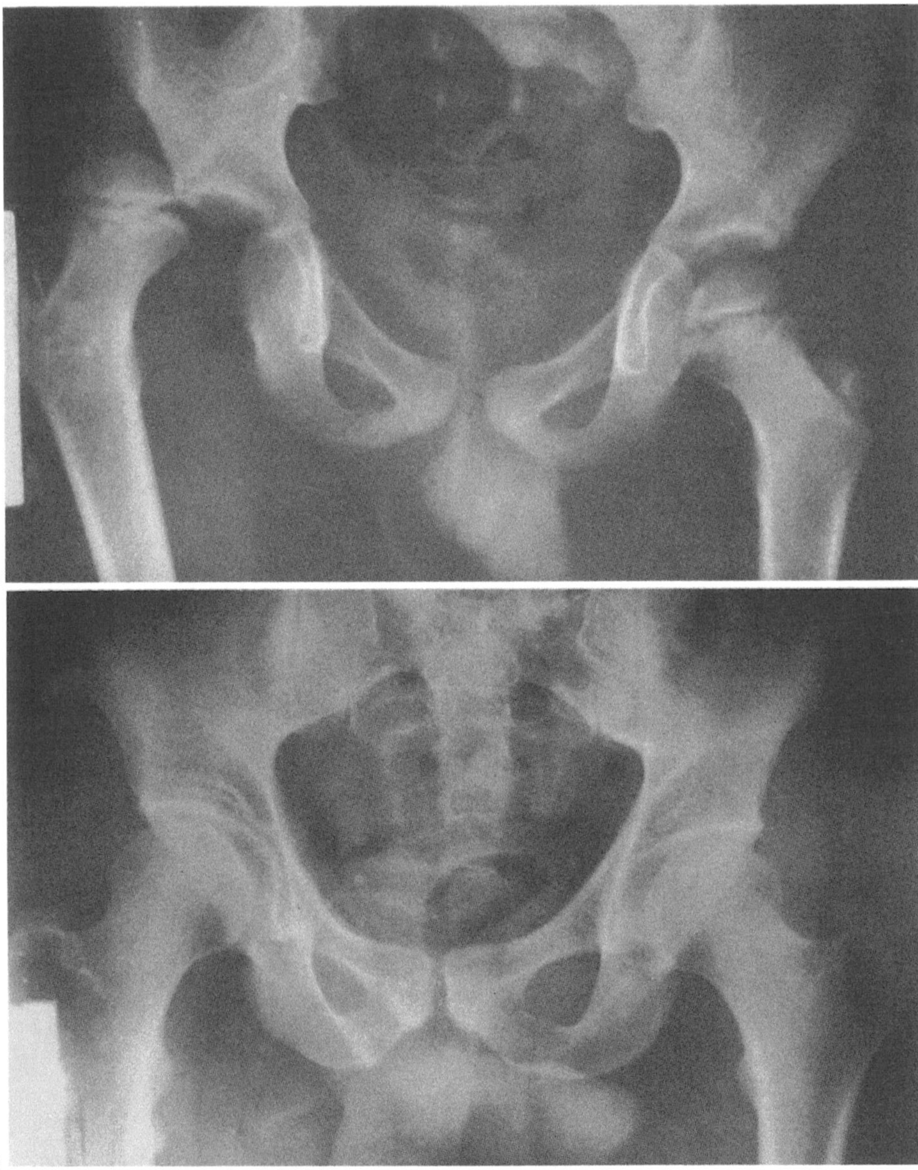

a

b

Fig. 3.4. **a** Iliac dislocation of the right hip in a 5-year-old boy who was pushed by another child while walking. Closed reduction was achieved 12 h later and a spica cast applied for 5 weeks. **b** Eighteen years later unrestricted activities, no pain, and normal morphology of the hip joint

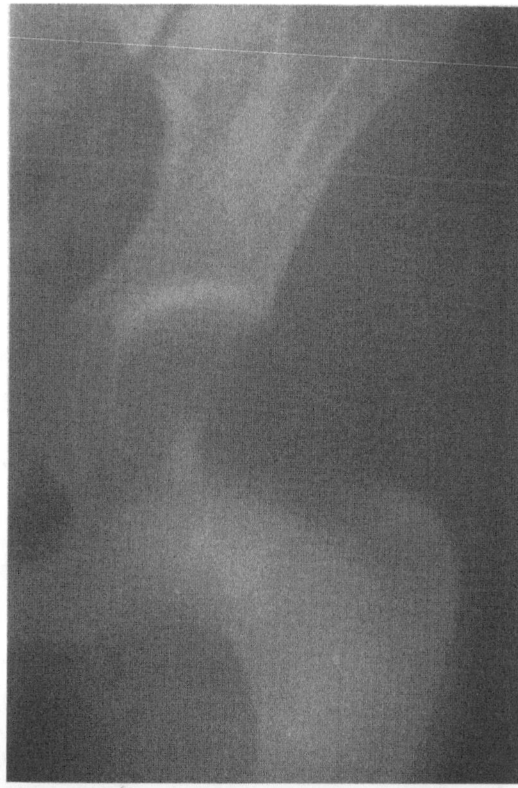

a

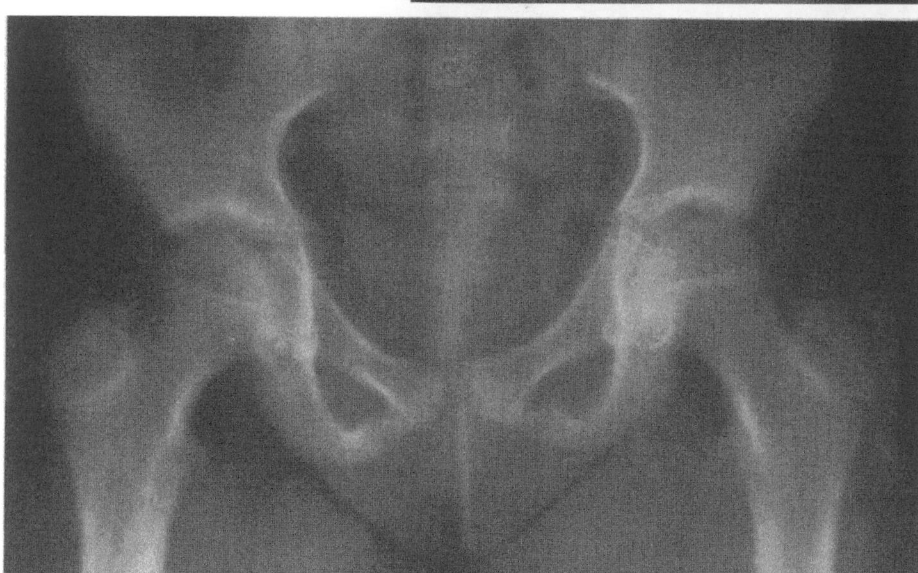

b

Fig. 3.5. **a** Ischiatic dislocation of the hip in a 10-year-old boy injured while playing football. Dislocation reduced by closed maneuvers within 6 h, and skin traction applied for 4 weeks. **b** At the latest follow-up, 3 years after the injury, the hip joint function and morphology are normal

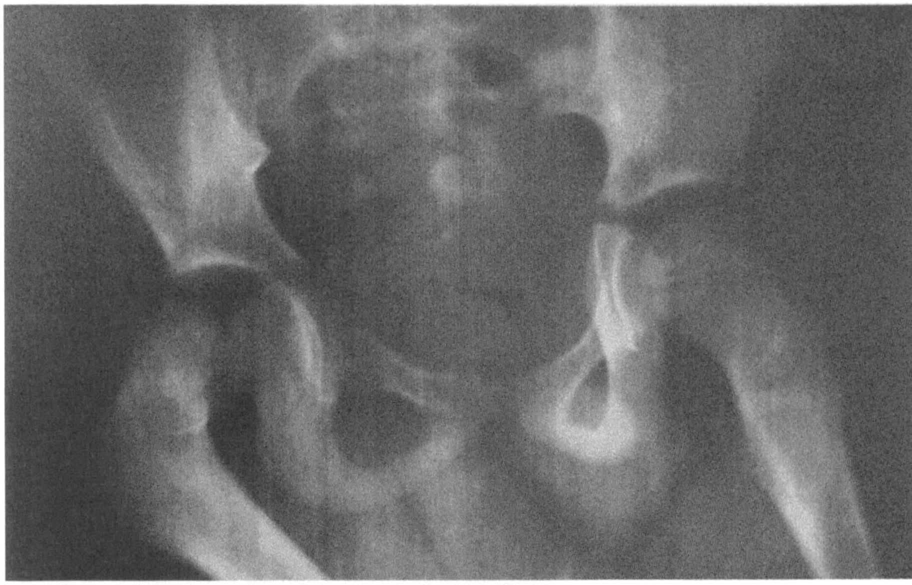

a

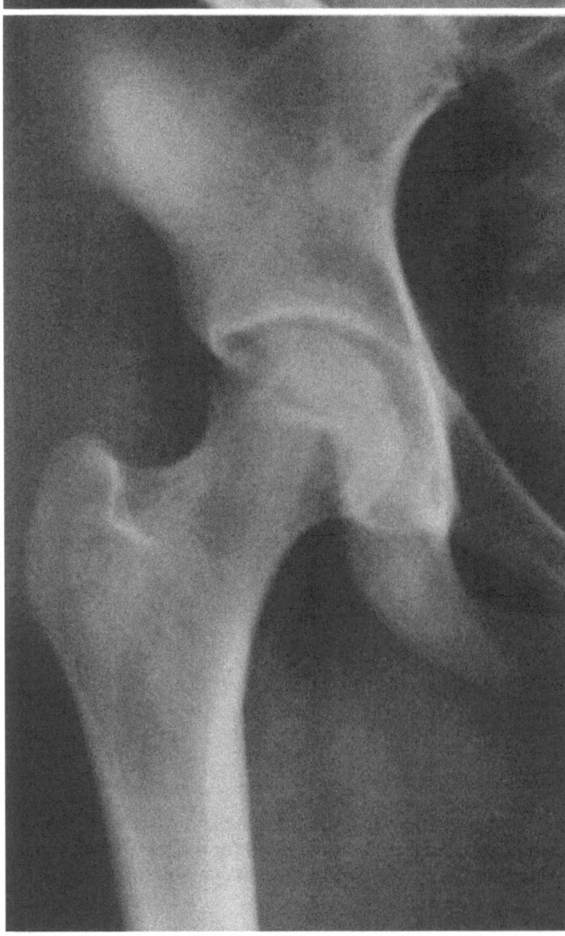

b

Fig. 3.6. **a** Retroacetabular right hip dislocation in a 9-year-old boy who tripped. Closed reduction was performed within 10 h, and a spica cast applied for 4 weeks. **b** Twenty years later the hip joint morphology and function were normal

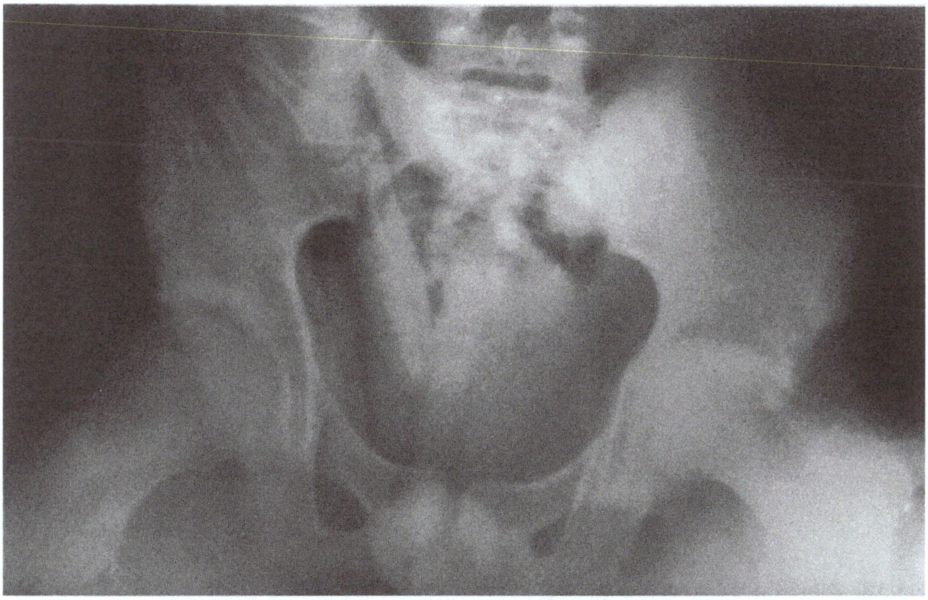

Fig. 3.7. Retroacetabular dislocation of the left hip in a 14-year-old girl, without lateral displacement of the proximal femur. The concentric projection of the luxated femoral head and acetabulum in the frontal roentgenogram may be responsible for diagnostic failure, which can be avoided by noting the different width of the medial joint space relative to the uninvolved hip

Ischiatic dislocations are low regular posterior dislocations. The femoral head is displaced posteroinferiorly and comes to lie at the base of the ischium or behind the tuberosity (Fig. 3.5). The limb is in adduction, internal rotation, and flexion. However, in ischiatic dislocations without altitudinal displacement, the femoral head lies immediately posterior to the acetabulum. These are so-called *retroacetabular* dislocations [21, 24, 109, 162, 486] (Fig. 3.6), which, in those cases where there is no lateral displacement, may cause incorrect diagnoses due to the concentric projection of the displaced femoral head and acetabulum in the frontal roentgenogram (Fig. 3.7).

Subischiatic dislocation is a low irregular posterior dislocation, with the femoral head being displaced under the ischium.

3.1.2 Anterior Dislocations

In anterior dislocations the femoral head is levered out of the acetabular socket through the anterior joint capsule [28, 146, 339, 351].

Pubic dislocations are high anterior regular dislocations. The femoral head is propelled either anterosuperiorly or directly anteriorly through this part of the capsule, coming to lie in front of the iliopubic column or in front of the anterior part of the acetabulum (Fig. 3.8). The limb is in abduction, external rotation, and extension. *Preacetabular* dislocations are pubic dislocations without altitudinal displacement.

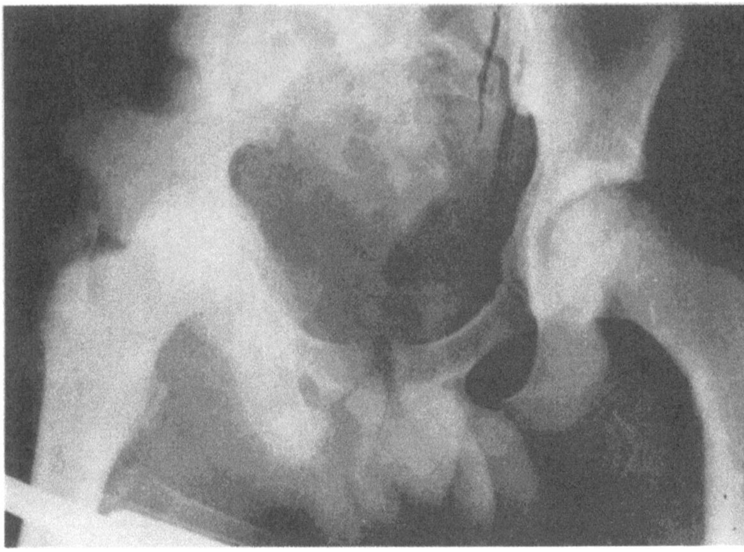

Fig. 3.8. Pubic dislocation of the right hip and bilateral fracture of ischial bone in a 15-year-old boy. (From Nerubay [339])

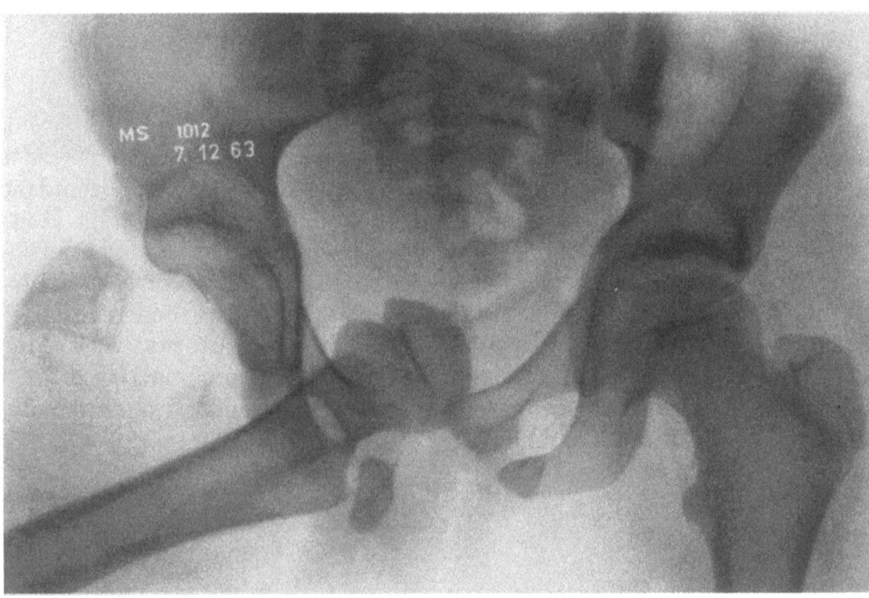

a

Fig. 3.9. **a** Intrapelvic dislocation of the hip, with associated avulsion of the greater trochanter, and fracture of the ipsilateral femoral shaft, in a 15-year-old boy. The dislocation was urgently reduced and internal fixation of the greater trochanter and the femoral shaft performed. **b, c** Condition 7 and 22 months later, respectively, showing avascular necrosis of the femoral head (of the adult type), with a sequester. **d** Eleven months later valguisation osteotomy with the purpose to change the weight-bearing sector of the head. **e, f** Two years after osteotomy: radiological stabilisation of deformity and fair functional result. (From Boitzy [53])

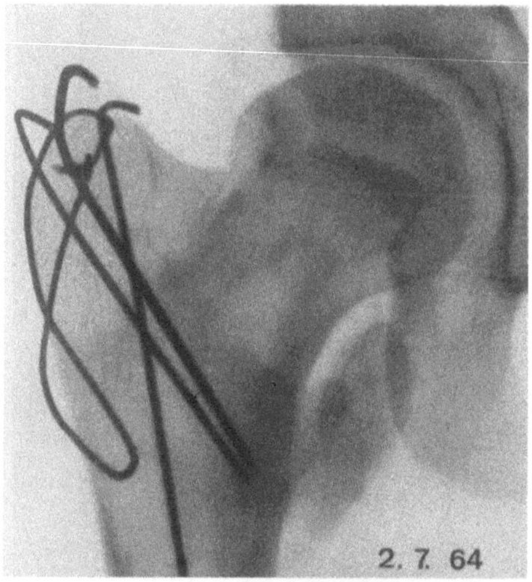

b

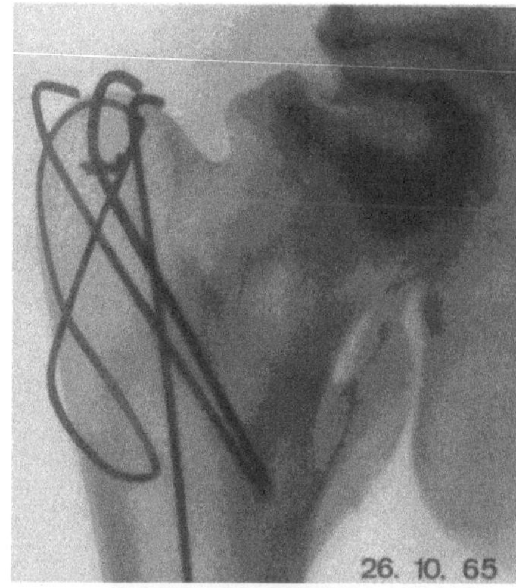

c

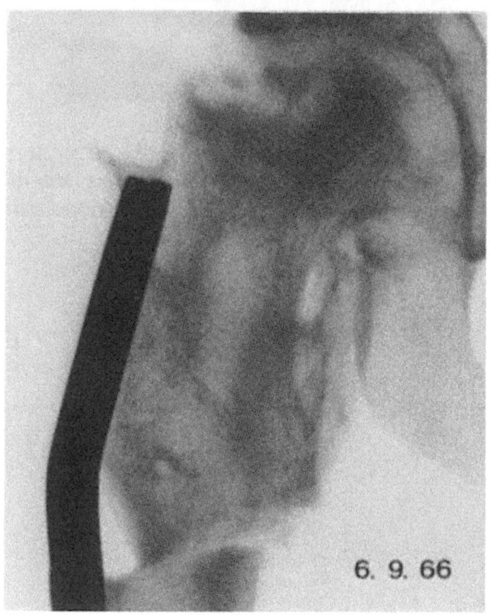

d

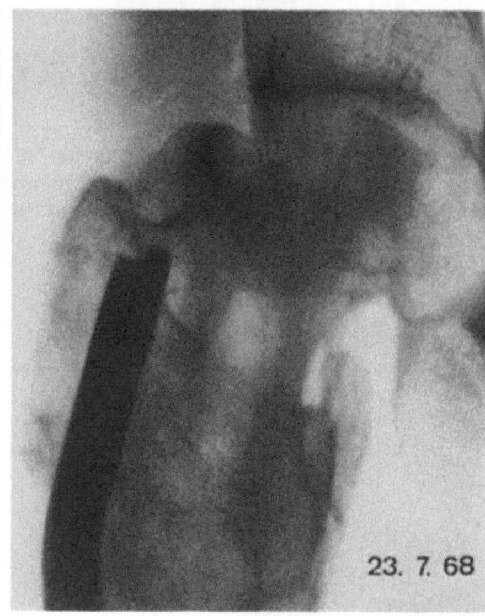

e

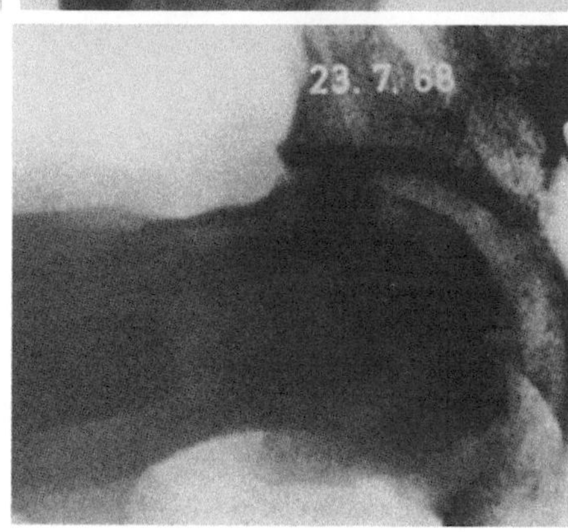

f

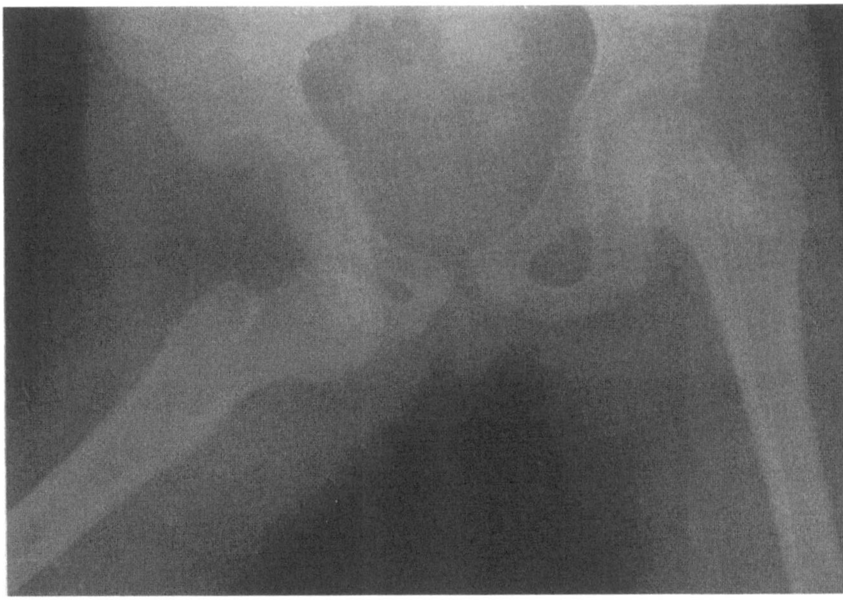

Fig. 3.10. Obturator dislocation of right hip in a 7-year-old girl injured while falling from a tree. Closed reduction was achieved 12 h later and a spica cast applied for 4 weeks. Four years later there was normal morphology of the hip joint and full pain-free range of motion and unrestricted activities. (From Barquet [28])

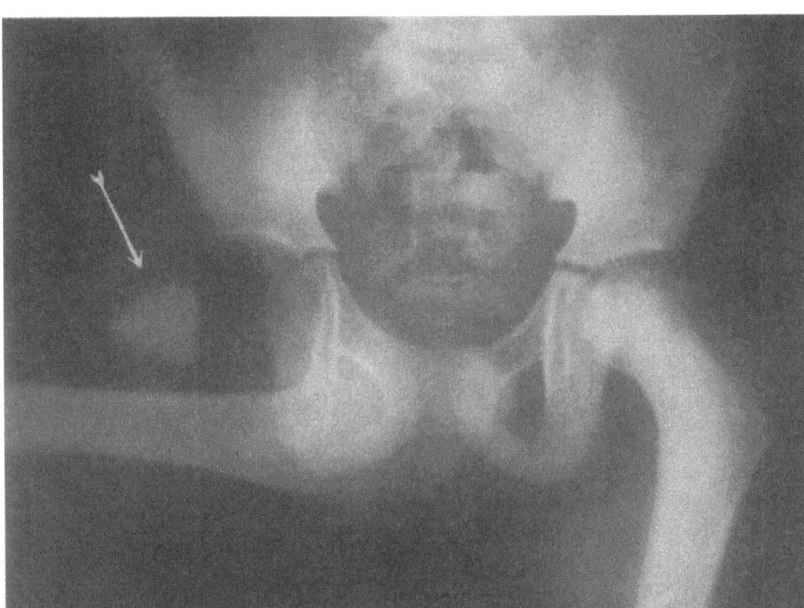

Fig. 3.11. Dislocation of the head of the femur into the scrotum and separation of the greater trochanter from the femur in a 10-year-old boy. (From Goetz [187])

There are, in addition, a variety of high anterior dislocations, such as *suprapubic,* with the femoral head resting over the pubic bone; *subspinous,* also called supracotyloid, with the head displaced so far upward that it comes to lie below the anteroinferior iliac spine; *anterior oblique,* with the head lying in front of the symphysis pubis [382]; and the so-called *intrapelvic* dislocation, where the head has been displaced along the horizontal branch of the pubis and comes to lie over the symphysis pubis, projecting "into" the pelvis (Fig. 3.9).

Obturator dislocations are low anterior regular dislocations. The femoral head is displaced through the front part of the joint capsule in an anteroinferior direction, coming to lie near the obturator foramen (Fig. 3.10). The limb is in an attitude of abduction, external rotation, and flexion.

Low anterior irregular dislocations are *perineal,* which is an extremely medially displaced form of obturator dislocation, the head lying in the perineum, and *scrotal,* with the head displaced even further, into the scrotum (Fig. 3.11).

3.1.3 Inferior Dislocations

In inferior dislocations the femoral head is dislocated below the acetabulum in the junction of the obturator foramen and the ischium, but with the femur in extreme flexion – the "erected" thigh touches the abdomen (Fig. 3.2). This condition is quite analogous to inferior dislocation of the shoulder.

3.1.4 Bilateral Dislocations

I prefer the criteria of Haudidier when classifying bilateral dislocations [215], and assign them as follows:

(1) Symmetric: bi-iliac (Fig. 6.1), bi-ischiatic, bipubic, and biobturator
(2) Assymmetric:
a. Armonic: iliac-ischiatic and pubic-obturator
b. Disarmonic: posterior (either iliac or ischiatic) and anterior (either pubic or obturator) (Fig. 2.2)

3.1.5 Incidence of Varieties

Most THDC are posterior [21, 46, 58, 98, 113, 146, 161, 172, 185, 230, 326, 329, 366, 370, 373, 407, 438, 471], with an incidence of 88.5% found in the WS. Furthermore, when comparing this incidence in children with the incidence of adult dislocations, as evaluated by several authors [57, 146, 281, 473], no difference can be found. Most posterior dislocations in children are iliac, 86.3% of the posterior dislocations in the WS. No significant differences have been found in adults relative to the incidences of iliac and ischiatic luxations.

In a 737-case series of THDA Epstein found a 12% incidence of anterior dislocations [146]. Similar findings have been presented in the literature [265, 281, 342, 467, 473]. A proportionately higher incidence of anterior dislocations in children than in adults has been considered a special feature of THDC [19, 184, 382]. However, Brug and Ziegelmuller reported an anterior dislocation incidence of 10% after reviewing 421 cases of previously reported THDC [58]. Among 923 THDC collected from the world literature, including 32 personal cases, I had found the incidence of anterior dislocations in children to be 12% [28]. Further evaluation of the WS confirmed this finding. Therefore, there is no difference in the incidence of anterior THDC, as with the incidence of posterior dislocations, between children and adults.

The incidence of obturator luxations has been considered to be proportionately higher in children than in adults [19, 101, 163]. Undoubtedly, obturator dislocations represent a higher incidence than the other varieties of anterior luxation in children (70%) [28, 113, 356, 412, 448]. However, if compared with the recorded series of anterior THDA [146, 281, 454], no significant difference concerning the incidence of obturator luxation can be found between adults and children.

Inferior dislocations are extremely infrequent, as only seven such cases in children have been collected [2, 121, 242, 314, 381, 407, 437], which gives an incidence of 0.5%.

In an attempt to provide comparative data, the incidences of the main varieties of THDC are presented as follows:

(1) Posterior Dislocations	88.47%
Iliac	76.33%
Ischiatic	12.14%
(2) Anterior Dislocations	11.53%
Pubic	4.22%
Obturator	7.31%

The difference in incidences of these varieties of THDC it is not arbitrary, but rather depends on the frequency of the pertinent pathogenic mechanisms for each variety of dislocation.

3.2 By Associated Lesions

3.2.1 Simple Dislocations and Fracture Dislocations

3.2.1.1 Simple Dislocations

Simple dislocations inherently produce certain soft tissue injuries, with the muscles in the pathway of the dislocating head being partially or completely torn or stretched. The *capsule* is torn either posteriorly or anteriorly, depending on the variety of dislocation. The tear is generally close to, or at the level of, the pelvic attachment of the capsule [74, 113, 288, 332, 351, 356, 381, 448], rather than near the thicker femoral attachment. The Y-ligament is rarely completely taut, except for the infrequent irregular dislocations. The *synovial membrane* is torn at the same site as the capsule and there is always hemorrhaging that, through the capsulosynovial tear, extends to the periarticular space [74, 356]. Although this hemorrhaging has been considered to be more severe in children than in adults [74, 327, 356, 381, 402], there is no reason or documentation substantiating this opinion. When a dislocation occurs, the *ligamentum teres* undergoes total rupture. Anyway the blood supply via the ligamentum vessels is of no significant value in the irrigation of the femoral head, as already shown. The injury to the *vessels supplying the proximal femur* will be considered in other chapters of this book. Severe lesions of the *periarticular muscles* are frequent in THDC, and according to several authors this is one of the differences between THD in children and adults [74, 113, 356, 381, 448]. However, here again there is no data supporting this statement.

Injuries to some other soft tissue structures may also occur. The *acetabular labrum* may be detached or torn in certain cases of posterior dislocation, eventually permitting its interposition between the cotyloid cavity and the femoral head when attempts at closed reduction of the luxation are performed, thus causing the irreducibility of the dislocation. Injuries to the *major vessels and nerves of the limb* may also occur and will be considered below.

Mild osteocartilaginous injuries, such as partial avulsions, minute fractures, and trabecular compressions, are considered to occur with a low frequency in THDC, and therefore, when present, may go undetected. However, avulsions may secondarily appear on the clinical scene because osseous or osteoperiostitic debris sometimes lead to heterotopic ossifications in the periarticular soft tissues, and also because the trabecular compressions at the femoral head may be responsible for certain trophic lesions, i.e., partial necrosis [236].

3.2.1.2 Fracture Dislocations

Associated fractures of the acetabulum and the proximal extremity of the femur determine a more severe grade of the dislocation, the so-called fracture dislocations (FD). Therefore, dislocations have been classified as simple dislocations, i.e., without joint fractures and FD.

FD of the hip are of low frequency in children [20, 21, 101, 103, 106, 163, 178, 244, 298, 324, 348, 351, 356, 370, 381]. Most of the longer published series [21, 101, 146, 253, 298, 348, 370, 441, 465] and the WS show the incidence of these FD to reach approximately 12%. Thus, most THDC are simple dislocations, i.e., 88%, making the ratio between simple luxations and FD 7:1, whereas in adults this ratio is approximately 1:1.8 [146, 148, 265, 400]. This is a basic fact differentiating THDC from THDA and deserves to be emphasized.

There are several reasons for this low incidence of FD of the hip in children: lower exposure to high energy trauma [178, 244, 413] and to those types of injuries usually causing THD in adults – for instance, dashboard injuries in automobile collisions are less frequent in young children, as their knees are below the dashboard level [107]; plasticity of the skeleton, where the abundant cartilage of the acetabulum and proximal femur, especially in young children, more easily absorbs and dissipates large forces [20, 101, 107, 178, 244, 324, 411, 424]; and greater capsuloligamentous elasticity, which allows the femoral head to separate from the acetabular rim at the moment of the dislocation, thus diminishing the impact [411, 424]. Milazzo and Fiandaca add an additional reason, stating that the acetabular socket in young children does not have the adult spherical shape, thus diminishing the risk of fracture of the posterior rim or wall, and also of the femoral head [324]. Furthermore, in addition to being infrequent, most of these FD occur in *older* children, with the presence of a lower proportion, of cartilaginous tissue, and greater forces dislocating the hip [12, 351, 376, 413].

FD of the hip in children may be classified as follows:

a) Dislocations with acetabular fracture
b) Dislocations with femoral head fracture
c) Dislocations with separation of the capital femoral epiphysis
d) Dislocations with femoral neck fracture
e) Dislocations with avulsion of the greater trochanter.

The most frequent associated fractures are those of the acetabulum, followed by the separation of the capital femoral epiphysis.

Dislocations with Acetabular Fracture. Although some authors have found a somewhat unexpectedly significant incidence of acetabular fractures in their series of THDC [70, 413, 420], most large series and the WS confirm a low incidence of this FD [21, 146, 172, 253, 298, 348, 370, 441]. The review of the WS, with 1440 cases of THDC, showed less than 90 cases with associated acetabular fractures [28, 55, 64, 70, 77, 78, 86, 146, 170, 178, 202, 224, 279, 283, 292, 298, 326, 356, 370, 376, 380, 381, 385, 413, 420, 427, 447, 465]. The incidence of these FD may be considered to lie between 7.5% and 8%. Those series with higher incidences of this fracture are mainly comprised of older children, with inherently higher frequencies of joint fractures.

These associated acetabular fractures occur in *posterior dislocations* in almost all instances. When, as a result of an indirect trauma, the femoral head is driven against the acetabulum, the head will either cause a fracture of the socket or, in exceptional instances, it will get fractured. These acetabular fractures correspond to the sector through which the femoral head has dislocated [65, 66], i.e., posterior acetabular rim, rim and floor, and diffuse fractures of the acetabulum including posterior and anterior columns in the most severe cases. The type of acetabular fracture associated with a dislocation is dependent on the position of the femur in relation to the pelvis at the moment of injury. The degree of adduction and flexion of the hip is a significant factor in different types of acetabular fractures. When adduction forces predominate, the head may be levered out of the socket to produce a simple dislocation. When longitudinal forces are greater than adduction forces, the femoral head is driven against the posterior acetabulum, leading to fracture of the socket. Acetabular roof fractures occur when longitudinal forces are applied to this part of the socket [4, 153].

The acetabulum represents an articular cavity of complex development, and is liable to be injured in children [113]. However, fracture separation involving the triradiate cartilage in association with a posterior dislocation is an exception and has been described only once [413]. However, FD of the hip in children mostly occur in older children, and in this age group growth cartilage is near definitive closure. Therefore, the biological condition in these children is most similar to that of adults, and an analogous method of classification can be applied. The criteria of Epstein [146] are very useful and recommended, as follows: (a) *Type 1:* with (or without) minor fracture – these dislocations with minor fracture are included in the same type

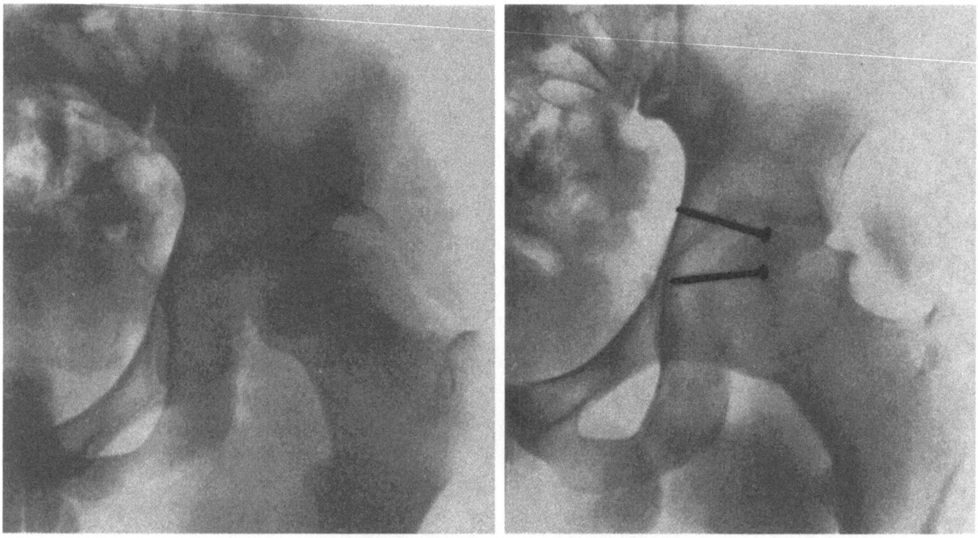

a b

Fig. 3.12. **a** Posterior dislocation with associated fracture of posterior acetabulum in a 15-year-old boy following a traffic accident. Immediate reduction of the luxation and reduction and internal fixation of acetabular fracture with two screws. **b** Mild radiological changes at the hip joint 4 years later. In spite of eventual mild pain, there is complete mobility of the joint. (From Rigault et al. [413])

as simple dislocations; *Type 2:* with a large single fracture of the posterior acetabular rim; *Type 3:* with a comminuted fracture of the acetabular rim, with or without a major fragment; and *Type 4:* with a fracture of the acetabular rim and floor.

Most posterior dislocations of the hip in children with associated acetabular fracture are those with minor fracture of the socket, i.e., type 1. A low percentage of cases correspond to type 2 injuries (Fig. 3.12). FD with a severe degree of damage to the acetabulum is very unusual in children, as shown by the WS (Fig. 3.13), while *anterior dislocations* with acetabular fractures are exceptional injuries.

Dislocations with Femoral Head Fracture. This severe FD, belonging either to the shear or to the compression type, is exceedingly uncommon due to the plastic, deformable, cartilaginous structure of the femoral head in children.

Few dislocations with *shear* fracture of the femoral head have been reported [44, 55, 146, 370, 414], with other associated fractures also present in some of them, e.g., separation of the capital epiphysis (Fig. 3.14) and acetabular fracture. These FD are *posterior* and may be classified, as in adults, according to Pipkin's criteria [386]: *Type 1* with femoral head fracture caudad to the fovea capitis femoris; *Type 2* with femoral head fracture cephalad to the fovea capitis femoris; *Type 3* types 1 or 2 with femoral neck fracture and, I would add, with separation of the capital femoral epiphysis; and *Type 4* types 1 or 2 with acetabular rim fracture.

THDC with associated *compression* fracture of the femoral head may occur when the head impinges on the anterior lip of the acetabulum as it moves outward in anterior dislocations [146, 236]. Recently, Jaberg and Ganz have emphasized this complex injury in anterior THDC [236], suggesting it might be more frequent than

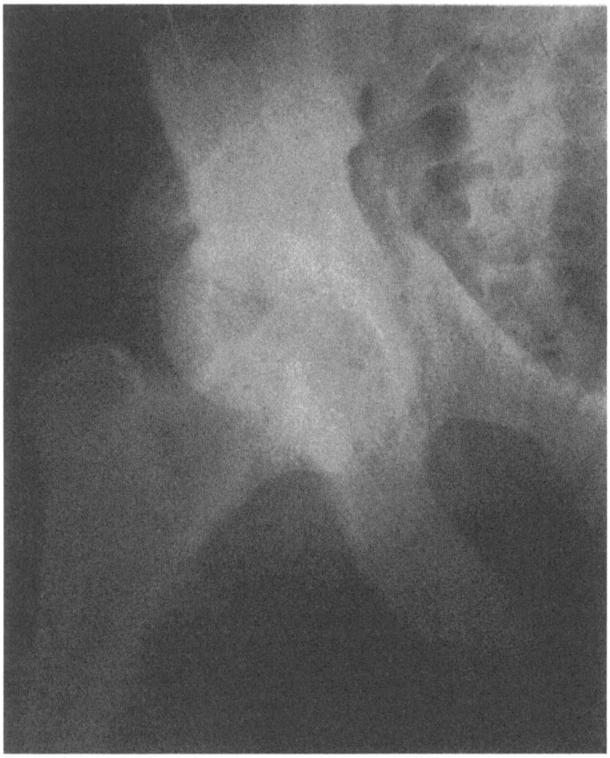

Fig. 3.13. Posterior dislocation of the hip with complete separation of the capital epiphysis from the femoral neck, i. e., combined injury type 1, and associated severe fracture separation of the acetabular columns in a 15-year-old boy following a traffic accident. Subsequently developed avascular necrosis, and hip arthrodesis was performed. (From Barquet and Vécsei [31])

previously considered. A compressive deformation of the femoral head would occur as a result of a ping-pong effect, with a fracture of the subchondral cancellous bone [51]. This compression effect would modify the surface of the femoral head in a small site or, in certain instances, a larger one (Fig. 3.15), with possible evolution of the compressed cancellous bone to segmental necrosis [236].

Dislocations with Separation of the Capital Femoral Epiphysis. This injury is the second most frequent among FD of the hip in children. A total of 33 cases were found in the WS [18, 31, 55, 62, 67, 71, 86, 129, 130, 160, 174, 179 a, 195, 271, 275, 283, 310, 368, 413, 427, 431, 436, 440, 446, 510].

Ekstrand and Tkazcuk [141] and Fiddian and Grace [159] reported on one and two cases of THDC, respectively, with no obvious initial separation of the capital epiphysis, but which, after reduction maneuvers, were recognized as dislocations with associated complete separation of the capital epiphysis. Doubts may arise as to whether separation had occurred initially and the displacement was dependent on manipulations, or if separation was strictly a consequence of manipulations.

a b

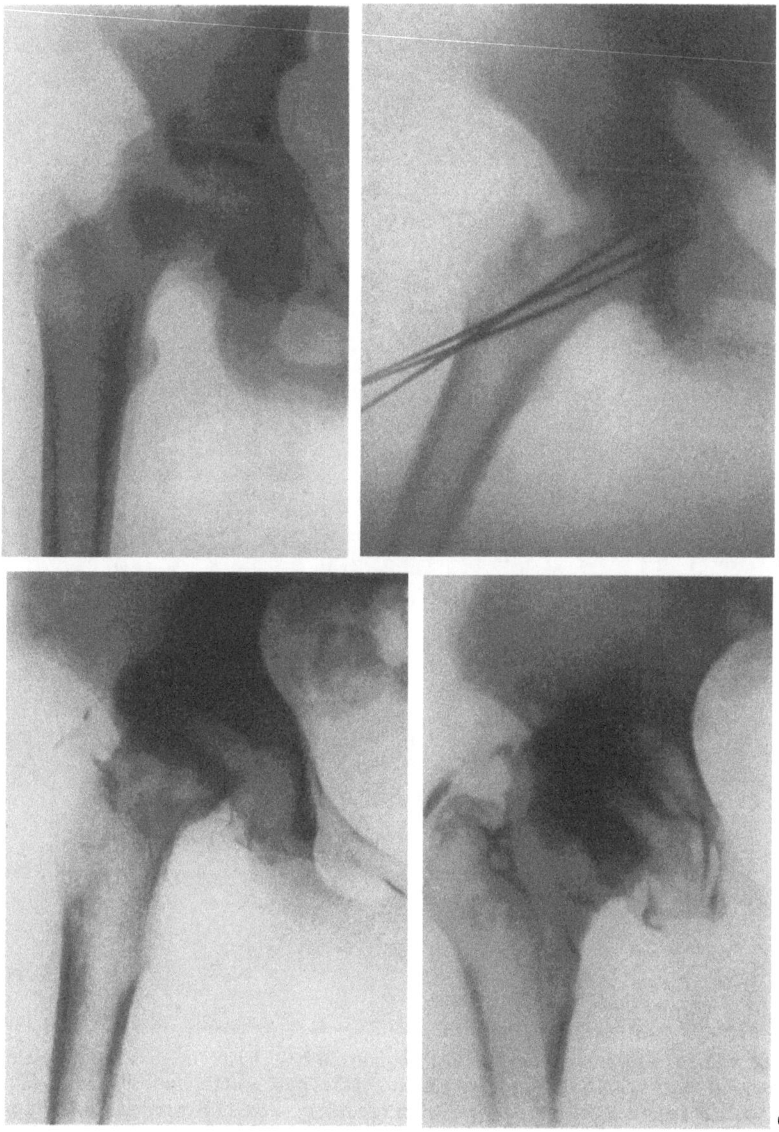

c d

Fig. 3.14. a Extremely severe complex injury to the hip in a 12-year-old girl – dislocation, shear fracture, and separation of the femoral head following a traffic accident. **b** Postoperative radiograph: open reduction and internal fixation of the major epiphyseal fragment to the femoral neck, and reduction of the dislocation; the small fragment of the femoral head has been removed. **c** Three months later: the femoral head has undergone complete resorption, the implants have been removed, and the acetabular socket is altered. **d** Two years later: there is a short and wide femoral neck, severe degenerative changes at the acetabulum, and limitation of hip mobility, together with severe limp. (From Bonvallet [55])

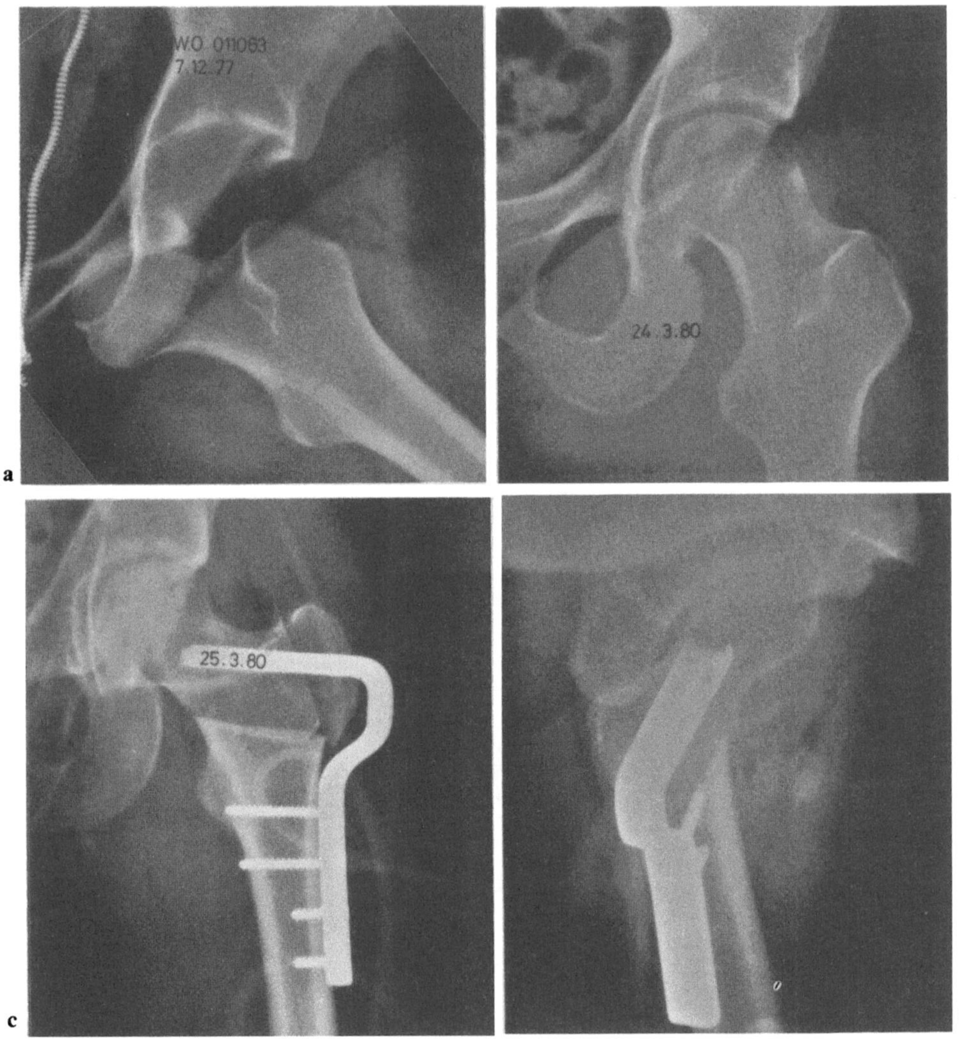

Fig. 3.15. **a** Obturator dislocation in a 14-year-old boy. **b** Anterolateral compression fracture of the femoral head. Within short-term evolution there is pain and limitation of rotation. **c** and **d** Intertrochanteric flexio-osteotomy 2¼ years after the injury. **e** and **f** Six months after surgery there is normal morphology and improvement of function of the joint. (From Jaberg and Ganz [236])

Whichever is the case, this event should be born in mind while reducing a "simple" THDC.

This type of FD, occurring in older children in more than 60% of the cases, seems to result from the application of two consecutive, but separate, severe forces to the hip [18, 31, 67]. The dislocation is the initial injury, since the forces would be exerted through the intact femoral neck. A second force then would lever the dislocated proximal extremity of the femur against the lateral aspect of the posterior acetabular wall and rim, leading to separation of the capital epiphysis.

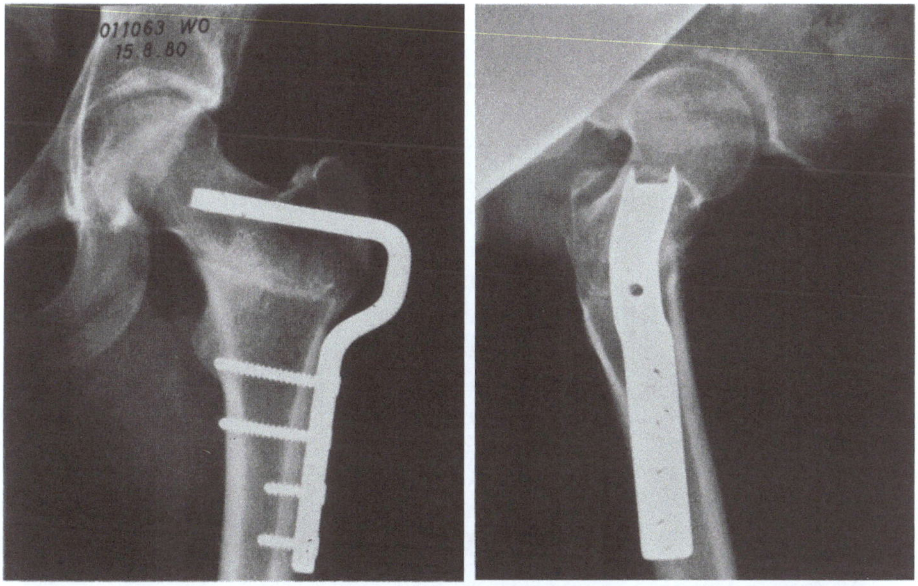

e f

Fig. 3.15

The separation of the epiphysis, also called transepiphyseal FD of the femoral neck, occurs through the region of hypertrophic cartilaginous cells and consists of a pure separation or a separation with fracture at the capital epiphysis. An associated fracture line through the metaphysis has not been found in the WS.

Concerning the pathoanatomy of this complex injury, two types have been described [31, 351]: *Type 1* with the capital epiphysis displaced out of the acetabulum and completely separated from the femoral neck (Fig. 3.16), and *Type 2* with dislocation of the capital epiphysis out of the socket and mild or moderate – but incomplete – separation of the capital epiphysis from the femoral neck (Fig. 3.17). The injury belongs to type 1 in most instances (94%), and there are associated fractures of the acetabulum in nearly 15% of cases.

Dislocations with Femoral Neck Fracture. This is an exceedingly rare FD of the hip in children, as only three such observations have been reported, two being posterior dislocations [202, 298] and one an anterior dislocation [160, 240] (Fig. 3.18).

This associated fracture is unexpected when the growth plate is still open [160]. The mechanism would be similar to that in dislocations with separation of the capital epiphysis [153, 259, 317, 375, 386]. The initial force dislocates the hip, and the second force levers the dislocated head against the iliac wing so that the femoral neck is fractured.

Dislocations with Avulsion of the Greater Trochanter. The incidence of avulsion of the greater trochanter in THDC should be emphasized, especially because this association of injuries has been rarely considered in the previous literature. Eleven such cases have been found in the WS that referred to anterior dislocations [53, 56, 69, 119, 137, 155, 187, 224, 351, 370], leaving one case for a posterior dislocation [258].

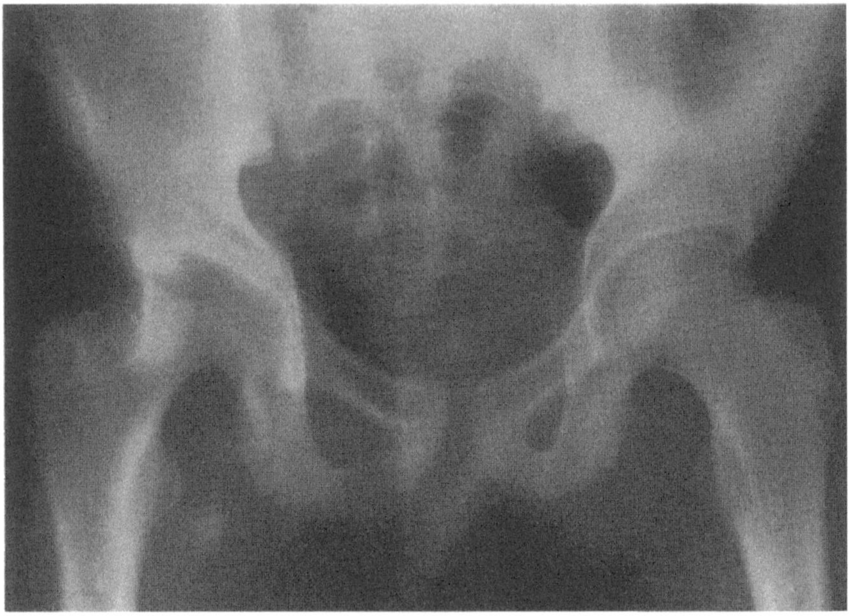

a

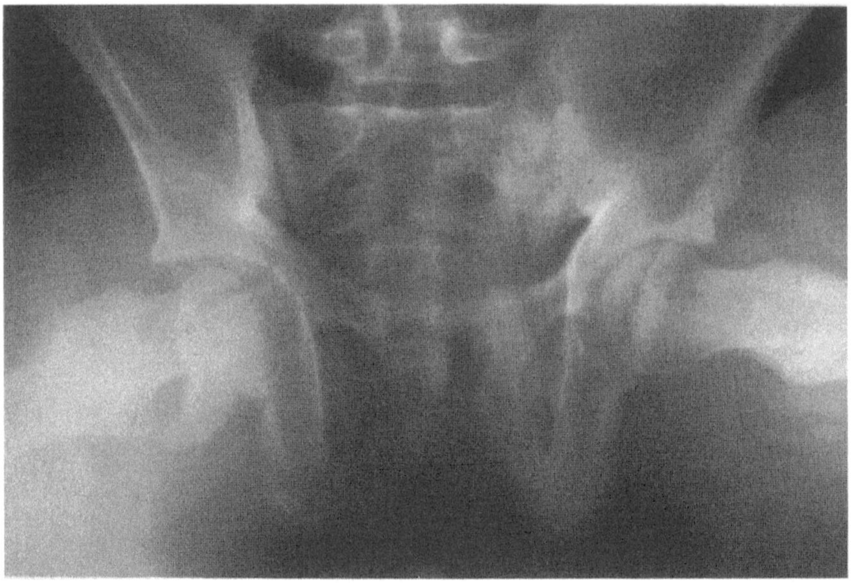

b

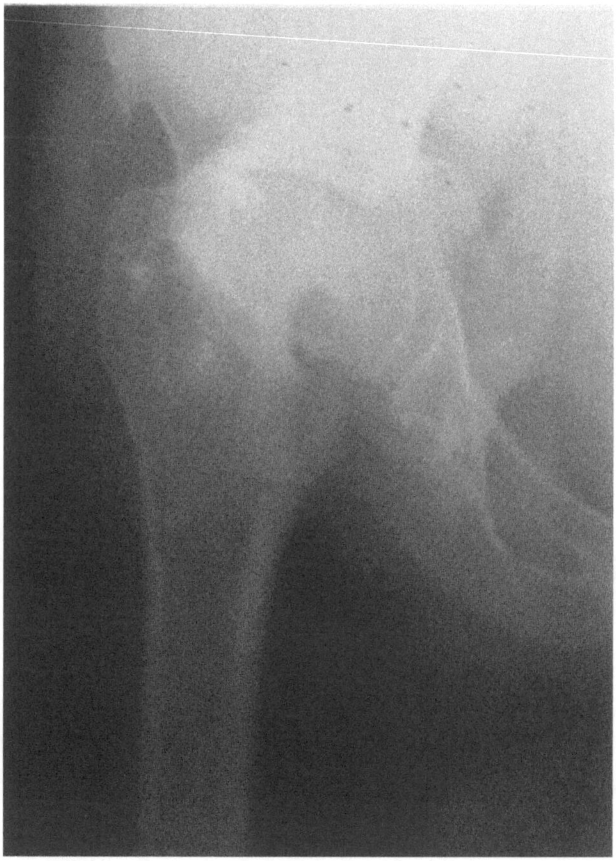

c

Fig. 3.16. a Anteroposterior view showing dislocation of the hip with separation of the capital epiphysis of the femur type 1, i.e., complete, in a 15-year-old boy who was struck by a car. **b** Roentgenogram with the hip in frog position, providing another view of the lesion. The initial therapeutic plan – open reduction and internal fixation – could not be performed due to severe thoracic injuries. Later on, removal of the epiphysis and an arthroplasty with interposition of fascia between neck and acetabulum was performed. **c** Anteroposterior view showing status of the hip 11 years after the injury; degenerative joint disease is severe. (From Barquet and Vécsei [31])

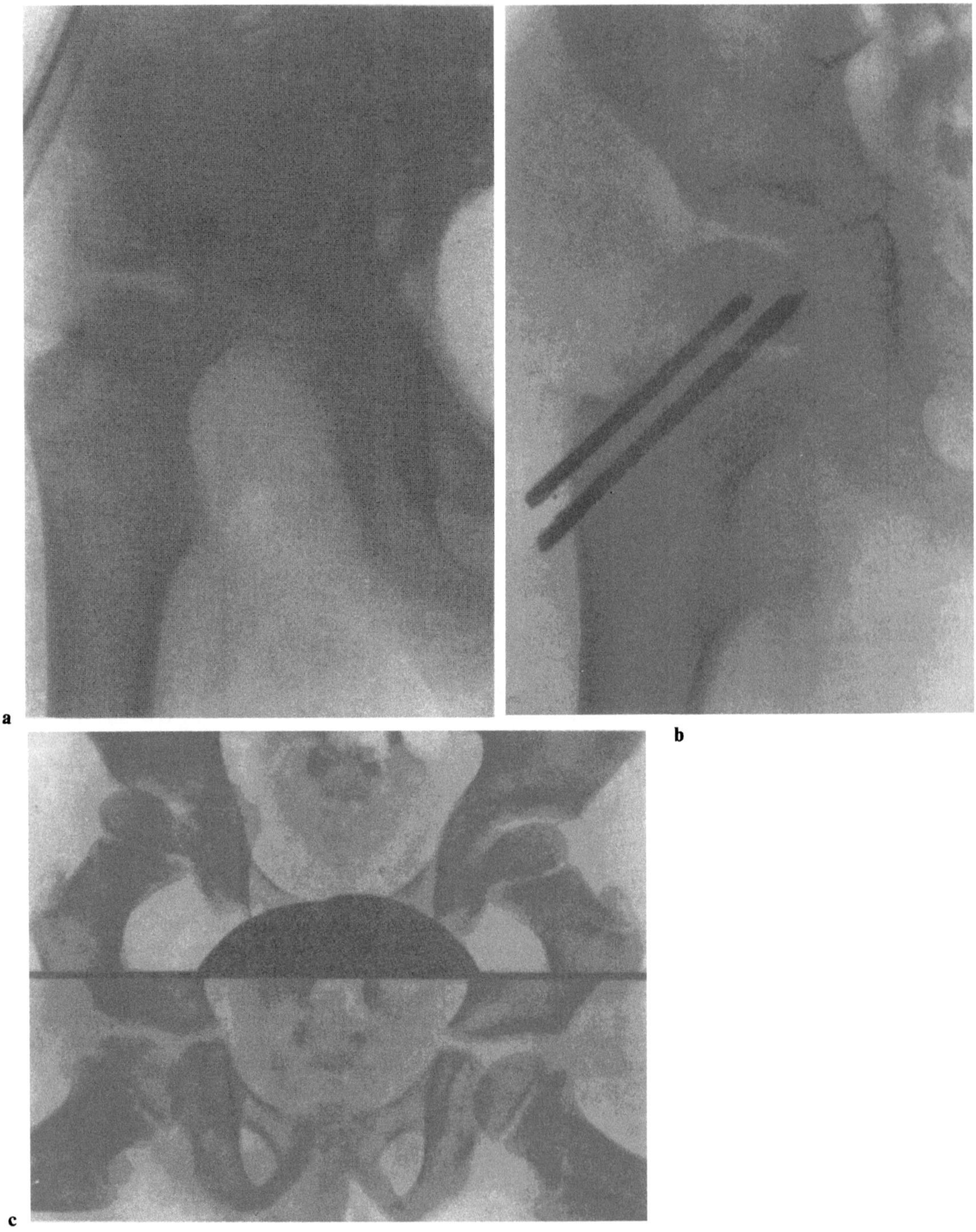

a
b
c

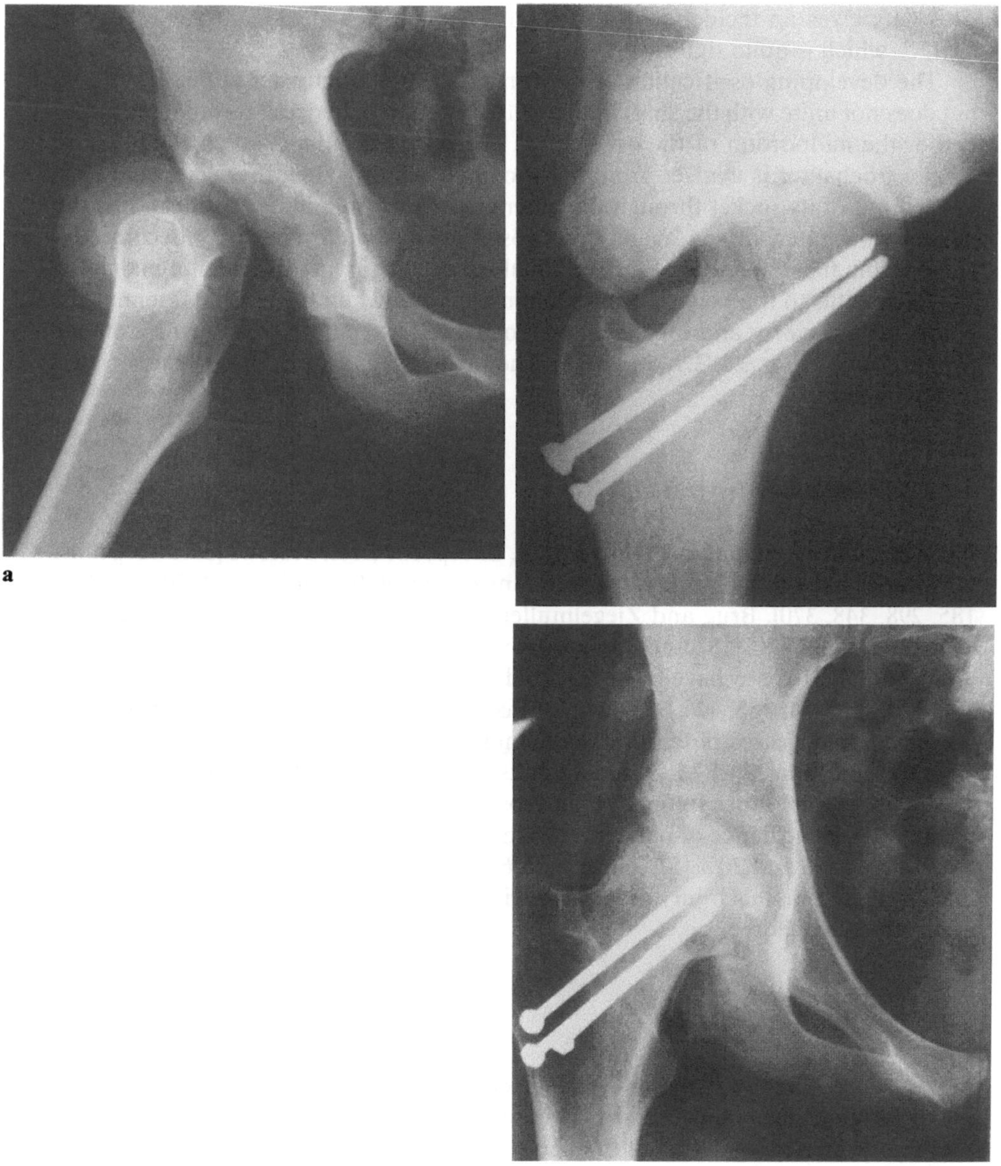

Fig. 3.18. **a** Girl (13 years 11 months old) with injured right hip: anterior hip dislocation with femoral neck fracture. **b** Early open reduction and internal fixation with two screws. **c** Seven months after injury there is evidence of avascular necrosis. (From Robertson and Peterson [420])

◁ **Fig. 3.17.** **a** Posterior dislocation of the right hip with incomplete separation of the capital epiphysis in a 4-year-old boy who was hit by a car. **b** Early open reduction and internal fixation of the proximal femoral unit with three smooth Kirschner wires. Later on the patient was placed in a 1½ spica cast for 10 weeks. **c** and **d** Two years after injury, anteroposterior and frog lateral views of the hip showing a viable femoral head and widening of the head and neck; there is full pain-free range of motion and unrestricted activities. (From Mass et al. [310])

This data gives an incidence of this lesion reaching 9% in the anterior variety of THDC, which is quite significant.

The developing ossification center for the greater trochanter appears at age 4, but does not unite with the shaft until age 18. Fractures can occur through the upper end or the midportion of the ossification center, but in almost all cases the entire greater trochanter is avulsed from the proximal femur. When the femoral head is levered out of its socket through the anterior capsule (in anterior dislocations) the greater trochanter, driven against the posterior acetabular rim, may become detached from the remainder of the proximal femur. The greater trochanter maintains its attachments to the pelvitrochanteric muscles, and when the proximal femur displaces far anteriorly and medially, the trochanter is separated a variable distance from its "bed" (Fig. 2.2, 3.9, and 3.11). The detachment may be pure or associated with a fracture.

*3.2.2 **Dislocations with Nerve Injuries***

Neurologic involvement in THDC is rare. Except for a few reviews [366, 420], most large series have shown its incidence to range between 0% and 4% [21, 70, 146, 172, 185, 298, 348, 370]. Brug and Ziegelmuller found the incidence to be 0.8% among 421 collected THDC [58], and the WS showed an incidence slightly over 2%.

Less than 30 cases have been reported [21, 70, 77, 111, 146, 298, 326, 328, 360, 366, 370, 420, 441, 465, 496, 513], with 26 instances of partial or total sciatic nerve involvement and 3 cases of femoral nerve injury. These nerve injuries occurred in 22 simple dislocations and 7 FD. As in adults, injuries to the peroneal element of the sciatic nerve were more frequent than those involving both the peroneal and tibial elements. The incidence of nerve involvement in THDA has been assessed as ranging between 4% and 20% [57, 146, 191, 256, 265, 281, 400, 473, 517], thus leading to the statement that this injury associated with THD is significantly more frequent in adults than in children.

3.2.2.1 Pathoanatomical Basis

Sciatic Nerve Injury in Posterior Simple Dislocations. Sciatic nerve deficiency in simple dislocations may be caused by peripheral nerve injury or by lumbosacral nerve root injury. Stretching, either of the nerve or of the nerve root, is the most common pathogenic mechanism in this type of dislocation. However, other authors have differed in the past as to the frequency of the site of injury. Sciatic palsy, while usually associated with FD in adult patients, has in most instances occurred in simple dislocations in THDC.

Nerve Stretch Injury. The close relationship of the sciatic nerve with the posterior aspect of the hip joint permits stretching of the nerve by the posteriorly dislocated femoral head [19, 20, 101, 107, 113, 163 356, 361, 400, 517]. As shown by Epstein, "the most important factor in the production of nerve injury in posterior simple dislocation may be the marked internal rotation of the dislocated hip, which causes a winding and tightening of the sciatic nerve" [146].

Different explanations have been given for the possibility of an isolated peroneal nerve palsy. Connolly considers the peroneal component of the sciatic nerve to be most susceptible to stretch by the dislocated head because of its oblique course, with less mobility than the tibial nerve, and also because the peroneal nerve has a greater number of axons in cross section and less intraneural fat for protection against trauma than those of the tibial nerve [87]. For Gregory, the greater susceptibility of the peroneal nerve is related to the valgoid relationship of the peroneal division to the piriform muscle. When the peroneal division passes through or above the muscle (12% and 0.5%, respectively), the nerve will be carried along and stretched, but this will not occur when the division passes below the muscle (87.5% of the cases) [191]. Gregory also states that when the displacement of the femoral head is far posterior, both divisions, peroneal and tibial, may be stretched [191]. Both Connolly [87] and Gregory [191] consider intraneural stretching as the usual mechanism of sciatic injury.

Lumbosacral Nerve Root Injury. As the stretch injury of the nerve does not seem to explain all facts in all circumstances [112, 382, 485], involvement of the nerve root has been considered as an alternative mechanism. On the basis of pathoanatomical, clinical and electromyographical facts, Decoulx et al. suggest that an injury to the lumbosacral nerve root would more frequently be the cause of sciatic deficiency in THD [112]. Protected by a resistant fibrous sheath, the nerve would escape compression, whereas the nerve root would be stretched or avulsed instead. This refers to the first sacral and the fifth lumbar nerve roots, and especially for the latter in a nearly vertical direction.

Decoulx et al.'s view, endorsed by Pidhorz and Mouterde [382] and by Traversa et al. [485], might explain the existence of sciatic palsy in posterior THD (with the nerve apparently uninjured), the isolated palsy of the peroneal nerve, and the rapid recovery of the tibial nerve deficiency in initial total nerve palsy with poor or no regression of the peroneal nerve palsy. Eisenberg et al. added evidence in favor of this pathogenic mechanism, showing avulsion of the lumbosacral nerve roots by means of myelography in clinical observations of neurologic deficiency associated with THD [140].

Sciatic Deficiency in Posterior FD. This condition in children may be the result of the above mechanisms, but also of stretching, direct pressure, or injury to the nerve by a detached acetabular fragment. These sharp fragments have been implicated in the genesis of sciatic nerve lesions in adults [146, 191, 517], but this is probably a rare cause of sciatic palsy in children. Nerve compression injury has been also implicated as a cause of secondary sciatic deficiency in FD [87, 191], related to entrapment of the nerve by scarring and callus formation occurring around the displaced acetabular bone fragments.

Femoral Nerve Deficiency in Anterior Dislocations. The lesion of the femoral nerve in THD results from stretching or pressing of the nerve by the dislocated femoral head, especially in pubic dislocation. However, this is an exceedingly uncommon associated lesion. No cases of obturator nerve palsy have been reported, as far as the WS shows.

Nerve Injuries During Reduction of the Dislocation. These injuries may occur, particularly when manipulations are difficult [281, 483]. Bigelow's circumduction procedure may also be considered responsible for sciatic nerve involvement [146].

3.2.3 Dislocations with Vascular Injuries

Damage to the femoral vessels in THDC, an exceedingly severe condition, has been considered extremely rare [54, 101, 304, 339, 382, 447]. Brug and Ziegelmuller [58] and Sterling and Meade [471] separately reviewed 421 and 492 infantile THD, respectively, from the literature and found the incidence of vascular involvement to be less than 1%. While reviewing the WS, nine such cases were found [54, 304, 339, 357, 370, 413, 447, 489], giving an incidence slightly over 0.6%.

This incidence has been assessed with both anterior and posterior dislocations being considered. However, damage to the femoral vessels in THD has been found only in anterior dislocations, and the incidence of this injury with respect to anterior dislocations in children is about 7%, indicating this is not a rare associated lesion. Fischer et al. indicated that these vascular injuries appear to be more frequent in children than in adults [163].

The pathoanatomical basis usually consists of vascular compression between the femoral head and the inguinal ligament [28, 54, 382] (Fig. 3.19). Compression or angulation of the artery, which occurs in most cases, may result in disruption of the intima and intramural hematoma or in intraluminal thrombus with occlusion [447], with the ensuing risks for each of these conditions. Section or laceration of one or both major vessels has also been reported [339, 447].

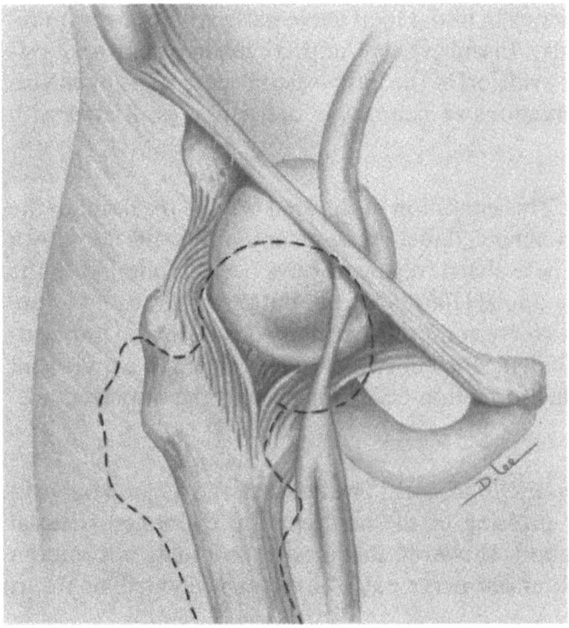

Fig. 3.19. Anterior dislocation of the head of the femur through the anterior capsule and iliofemoral ligament, with compression of the femoral artery against the inguinal ligament. (From Bonnemaison and Henderson [54])

3.2.4 *Dislocations with Ipsilateral Femoral Shaft Fracture*

THDC with ipsilateral femoral shaft fracture (IFSF) are rare. Forty-six such cases were found in the WS [21, 25, 44, 53, 70, 84, 88, 103, 146, 148, 151, 170, 185, 188, 214, 218, 227, 252, 291, 295, 304, 313, 315, 360, 385, 390, 413, 415, 426, 441, 442, 443, 454, 456]. The incidence of this associated lesion in children is approximately 3.6%, which is similar to the incidence of this condition in adult dislocations [57, 146].

Hip dislocation is posterior (Fig. 3.20) in 80% of cases, and anterior (Fig. 3.21) in 20%, a figure which might suggest that the incidence of dislocation with IFSF is somehow proportionately greater in anterior than in posterior pediatric hip dislocation, considering the incidence of each of these varieties.

Since Kammerer [252], most authors have agreed that this associated injury is the outcome of two consecutive, but separate, traumatic events [25, 107, 218, 304]. The dislocation would be the first injury. A second force, acting directly and at right angles to the femoral shaft, already with impaired mobility as a result of the dislocation, would produce the shaft fracture [25, 218, 304]. The shaft fracture is more or less transverse in most cases, the fracture line predominating at the middle third of the shaft.

On the other hand, Alho has reviewed a series of ipsilateral hip dislocations (and fractures) and femoral shaft fractures, concluding that with axial loading lineal or comminuted femoral shaft fractures occur simultaneously with the dislocation [4]. Similar opinions have also been presented [6, 30a, 409, 417]. Thus, THD and IFSF may also be combined injuries caused by massive axial loading to the femur.

The usual etiology of this combination of lesions, such as traffic accidents or falls from heights, supports both previously considered mechanisms, which I also believe are involved in the pathogenesis of this association of injuries.

3.2.5 *Open Dislocations*

In exceptional cases the hip suffers an open dislocation, a condition which applies to both children [101, 163, 415] and adults [196]. Reports of open luxations of the hip are seldom for children [15, 119, 120, 193, 348, 413, 415, 447]; an incidence of 0.5% may be estimated. These are usually extremely displaced anterior dislocations. The soft tissue injuries are extremely severe, and may include damage of the femoral vessels. This, together with the increased risk of infection, makes the prognosis of this injury extremely poor.

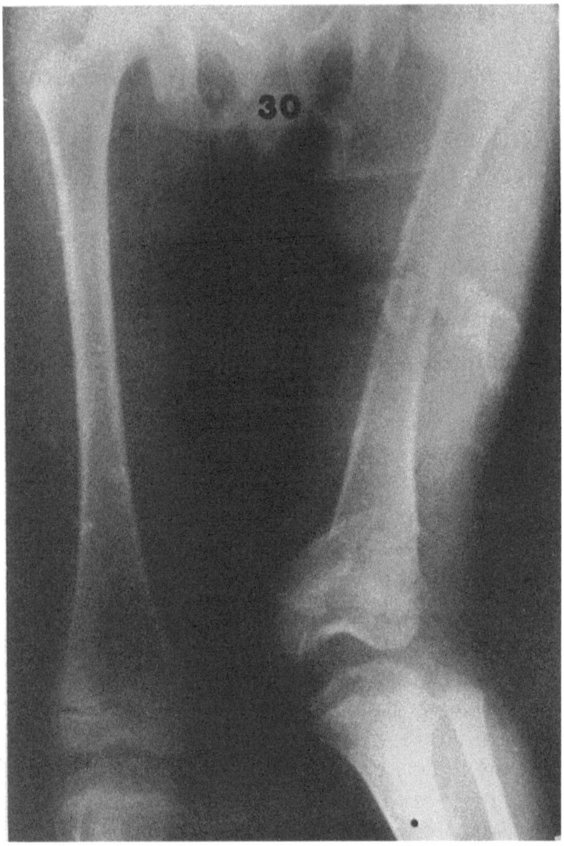

a

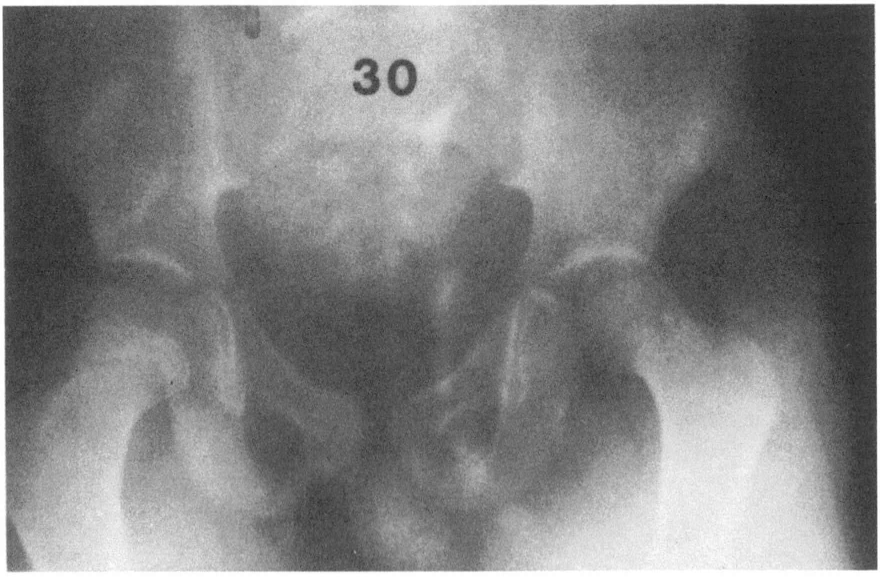

b

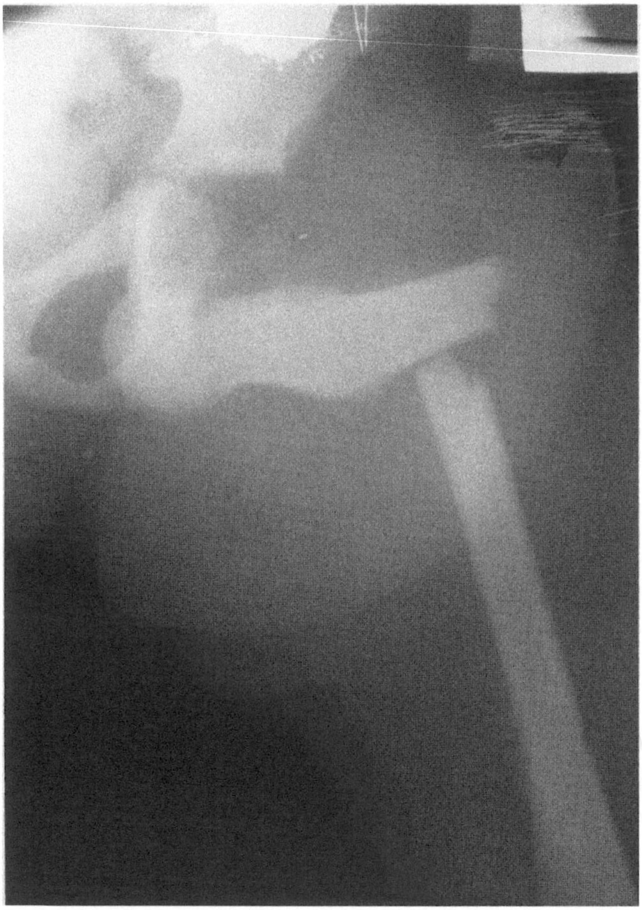

Fig. 3.21. An exceptional case of obturator dislocation of the hip, associated with ipsilateral fracture of the femoral shaft in a girl of 6 years. (From Barquet [21])

◁ **Fig. 3.20.** **a** Radiogram showing transverse supracondylar fracture of the left femur in a 4-year-old boy who was struck and driven forward by a motor vehicle. The abnormal attitude of the proximal fragment in adduction and internal rotation were initially missed. **b** Anteroposterior X-ray of the pelvis showing a posterior dislocation of the left hip with very mild upward displacement. (From Barquet [25])

4 Recent Dislocations

4.1 Clinical Features

The child is frequently brought to the hospital by his parents or by people who were nearby when the accident took place. Useful information may thus be obtained concerning the causative trauma – severity, mechanism, etc. – and in the case of the child's parents, a clinical history of possible previous afflictions of the hip joint. The frequency of trivial trauma in the genesis of THDC should be emphasized, in order that the orthopedic surgeon bears in mind the possibility of THD in these instances.

4.1.1 Symptoms and Signs

The basic clinical pattern of THD is similar in children and adults; age is not a differential factor in this regard [19, 74, 101, 103, 243, 329, 411, 413, 424, 483].

The child is in pain and active movements of the injured hip joint are completely restricted. The child holds its painful thigh still and resists passive motion [107]. Nevertheless, although constant, these symptoms vary in severity [20, 500].

As in adults, a child having suffered a THD displays a typical clinical pattern with respect to the injured limb, which is sufficient to allow not only the diagnosis of hip dislocation, but also the variety (Fig. 4.1).

In posterior dislocations the involved thigh is held in adduction and internal rotation. Flexion is significant in ischiatic dislocations and mild in the iliac variety, simulating extension when the patient is in dorsal decubitus, as a result of compensating lordosis. The limb is extended in high iliac dislocations. There is also resistance to passive external rotation and abduction in posterior dislocations. As shown in Chap. 3a, Monteggia's dislocation occurs with the leg adducted, flexed, and everted.

With anterior dislocations the hip is held in abduction and external rotation; there is flexion in the low variety, i. e., obturator, and extension in the high variety, i. e., pubic. The amount of abduction in anterior dislocations is variable and depends on the degree of displacement of the head along the pubic ramus or the obturator foramen: the farther it lies medially, the greater the abduction of the thigh. Passive adduction and intrarotation are impossible.

An inferior dislocation (Fig. 3.2) occurs with the hip acutely flexed; the "erected" thigh contacts the anterior abdominal wall. The hip may be slightly adducted or abducted, or in a neutral position between adduction and abduction, and usually in neutral rotation.

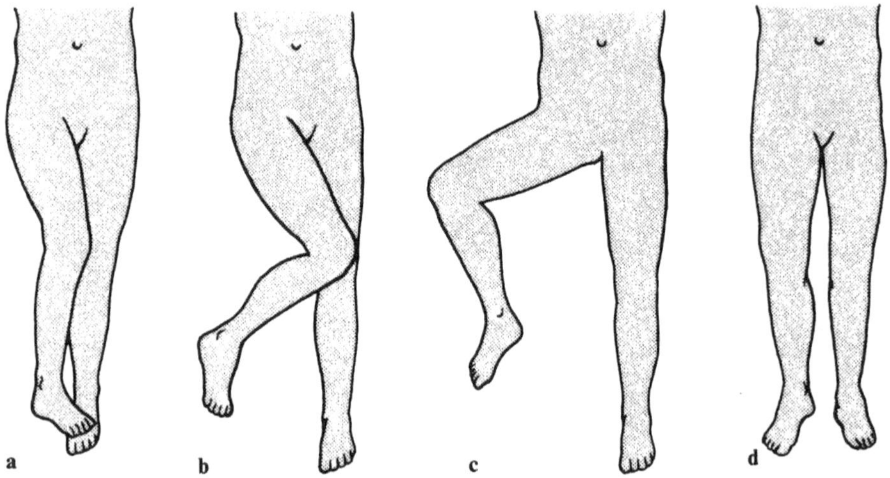

Fig. 4.1 a–d. Typical deformity of the lower limb in the main varieties of traumatic hip dislocation. **a** Iliac; **b** Ischiatic; **c** Obturator; and **d** Pubic

Shortening of the limb is found in posterior iliac dislocations. However, apparent or even true lengthening has been described in obturator dislocations [91, 101, 113, 184, 399, 467]. Nevertheless, length measurements of the lower limbs are unreliable and fortunately not necessary for diagnosis.

The femoral head is often palpable in its new position, an additional clinical sign of THD. In posterior dislocations palpation in a thin patient may permit the examiner to feel the head beneath the gluteal mass or near the ischium, but when there is much subcutaneous fat it is impossible to adequately palpate the head [467]. In front of the joint the normal fullness caused by the presence of the head below Poupart's ligament is lacking, and a finger can be depressed into the tissues.

With anterior dislocations, there is femoral head prominence at the groin, below Poupart's ligament in pubic dislocation, while in the obturator variety the head of the femur can sometimes be palpated toward the thyroid depression, in the adductor muscles compartment. In irregular anterior dislocations the head is sometimes palpated according to its definitive position, below the anteroinferior iliac spine, in front of the symphysis pubis, in the perineum, or in the scrotum. Whichever the anterior luxation, there is always a lack of normal prominence of the greater trochanter.

Whenever these examining steps are followed, it will be possible to easily achieve a clinical diagnosis of hip dislocation, including the variety. However, it should be remembered that when the injury to the child, and especially one in the younger group, has resulted from a trivial accident, the dislocation may be missed initially if the examination is not adequate, but also because the child may not permit a correct examination [382].

The knee will frequently show evidence of direct trauma to its anterior aspect: a visible laceration, abrasion, contusion, or even fracture. The knee should always be thoroughly examined to rule out an associated injury, due to the pathogenic mechanism of THD.

4.1.2 Special Circumstances

Certain circumstances in which the early diagnosis of THD is at high risk should be underlined.

In the Multiply-injured Child. The child is usually in shock, and the other significant injuries (encephalic, thoracic, abdominopelvic, or at the limbs) may distract one's attention from the hip lesion [63, 68, 111, 263, 382, 385, 438, 500], especially because these are life-threatening lesions, but also because there is a low index of suspicion due to the rarity of THDC [25, 151]. Delayed diagnosis often occurs in multiply-injured children. Thus, every child with multiple injuries must be carefully evaluated in order to avoid missing a THD.

THD with Associated Ipsilateral Femoral Shaft Fracture (IFSF) (Figs. 3.20 and 3.21). While reviewing the WS, I found in 43% of the THD with IFSF that the dislocation went unrecognized initially, diagnosis being performed between 3 days and 24 months, after an average of 5 months [25]. This high incidence of missed diagnoses has been indicated in pediatric THD by other authors [63, 103, 107, 151, 351, 385, 413, 506]. Other papers, mostly referring to this associated injury in adults, have presented similar findings [114, 139, 218, 296, 400, 442]. It is interesting to note that if the dislocation is not diagnosed within the first few days, then it remains unnoticed until difficulties are encountered in alignment of the femoral fracture in traction, or until the patient starts to walk after the femoral fracture has healed [25, 218, 442]. There are several reasons leading to the failure to diagnose the hip dislocation: (a) the examiner is confronted with a major and obvious deformity, the femoral shaft fracture, which appears to explain the clinical situation and distracts the attention from the lesion of the hip [25, 103, 151, 218, 295, 386, 442]; (b) the attitude of the lower limb characteristic of the dislocation is absent, and the fracture, acting as a corrective osteotomy, removes the signs of the hip dislocation [25, 63, 151, 218, 415, 442]; and, as previously stated (c) the possibility of a hip dislocation, being an infrequent injury in children, is usually not present in the mind of the attending surgeon [25, 151].

Several procedures have been recommended in order to avoid overlooking the diagnosis of hip luxation in this associated injury. A thorough clinical examination of the hip has been advised as routine to detect certain signs which indicate a hip dislocation in every patient with a fracture of the femur, including elevation of the greater trochanter, posterior prominence of the femoral head, and buttock bruising in the case of posterior dislocations; and, in anterior dislocations, femoral head prominence in the inguinal area and loss of the normal prominence of the greater trochanter [218, 506, 517]. However, these signs are difficult to recognize in a child in pain and frequently in shock, and they can be masked by swelling in the hip region, which is a normal feature of many femoral shaft fractures [25, 151]. As will be shown below, the diagnostic clue in these instances is radiological.

4.1.3 Associated Nerve Injuries

The need for a thorough neurological examination of the lower limb in cases of trauma to the hip is classic. By these means, the orthopedic surgeon will search for neurological deficiency, which may eventually be precisely defined with electrical examinations. Although uncommon, this associated lesion must be especially considered from the standpoint of prognosis and treatment.

The clinical differences between nerve injuries and nerve root injuries are somewhat difficult to demonstrate. However, a meticulous neurological examination provides certain clues in the differential diagnosis. An electromyographical examination performed 3-4 weeks after the injury may also add information in order to achieve a definite diagnosis [112, 382].

4.1.4 Associated Vascular Injuries

A clinical evaluation of the circulatory status of the affected limb is indispensable. However, this evaluation may be hampered by unconsciousness, by inadequate perfusion secondary to shock, or by severe fractures and dislocations [447]. Nevertheless, the slightest suspicion of inadequate perfusion of the limb requires special diagnostic measures, and sometimes certain therapeutic procedures should be urgently performed.

4.2 Roentgenographic Diagnosis

The clinical examination is to be immediately followed by an adequate and complete radiological examination, which is essential not only for the definite diagnosis of hip dislocation (usually confirming the initial clinical diagnosis), but also for the type of dislocation, i.e., whether it is a simple dislocation or a FD.

Some authors assume that an anteroposterior radiological view is usually satisfactory for diagnosis. Undoubtedly, gross displacements of the femoral head of the dislocated hip are evident on X-rays. However, the isolated use of an anteroposterior view may lead to severe diagnostic pitfalls in subtler displacements [191], especially in retroacetabular dislocation. In this latter variety, standard frontal roentgenograms may show a seemingly normal "concentric" projection of femoral head and acetabulum (Figs. 3.7 and 4.2) [21, 24, 101, 103, 109, 162, 486], and even though there is also a femoral rotation, sometimes it is not possible to detect this rotation, especially because it is not possible to detect the lesser trochanter, which does not ossify until adolescence [350].

Whenever confronted with a THD, a radiological view of the contralateral hip must be performed. A simple frontal view of the pelvis is inexcusable, as both hips should be compared (Fig. 3.7): Shenton's line, roof-head congruity, and comparative dimensions of the femoral heads [191]. The interruption of Shenton's line indicates that the hip joint is disturbed. The variance in dimensions of the cartilaginous space on the injured hip joint as compared with the contralateral one suggests abnormal displacements of the head. The disparity of femoral head dimensions confirms the suspicion of a dislocated hip.

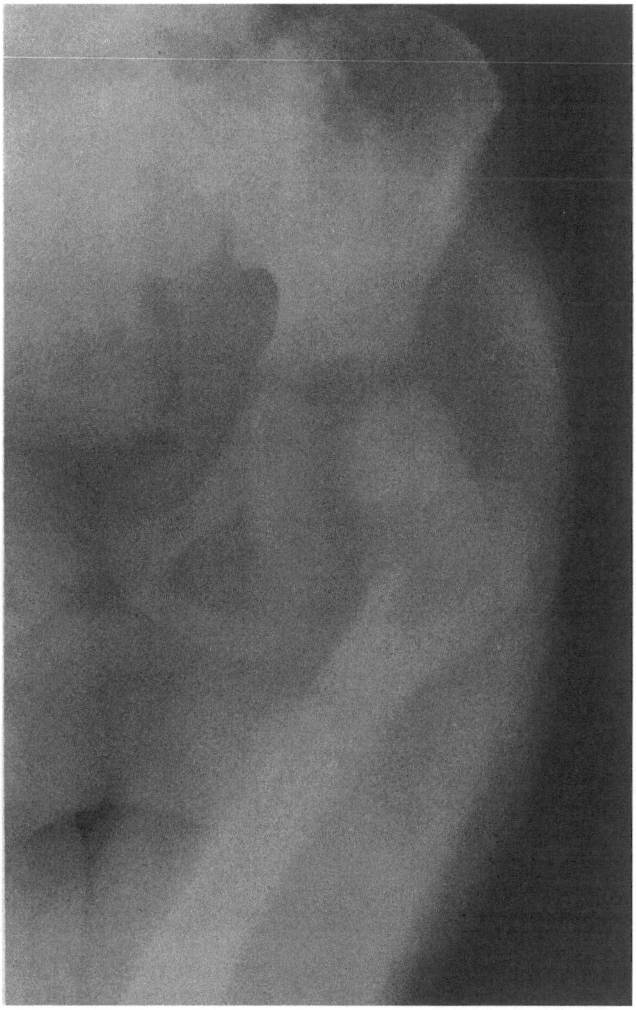

Fig. 4.2. Posterior retroacetabular dislocation of the left hip in a 9-year-old boy, who fell while running and was fallen over by another boy. Frontal radiographic view: note the concentric projection of femoral head and acetabulum

An adequate radiological examination should be performed with at least two views. A true cross-table lateral view of the hip should also be routinely performed in dislocation injuries of the hip joint, in order to contribute to diagnosis [21, 24, 101, 103, 162, 486] (Fig. 4.3). I would insist upon this since, while reviewing 24 posterior THDC, six retroacetabular dislocations were found, one of which was initially missed in spite of an adequate frontal roentgenogram [21].

Confronted with FD of the hip, the anteroposterior view shows the position of the anterior and posterior columns, the medial wall and roof of the acetabulum, and also the acetabular posterior and anterior rims. However, this view has no depth, and even though it may indicate that there is an acetabular fracture, there is no good

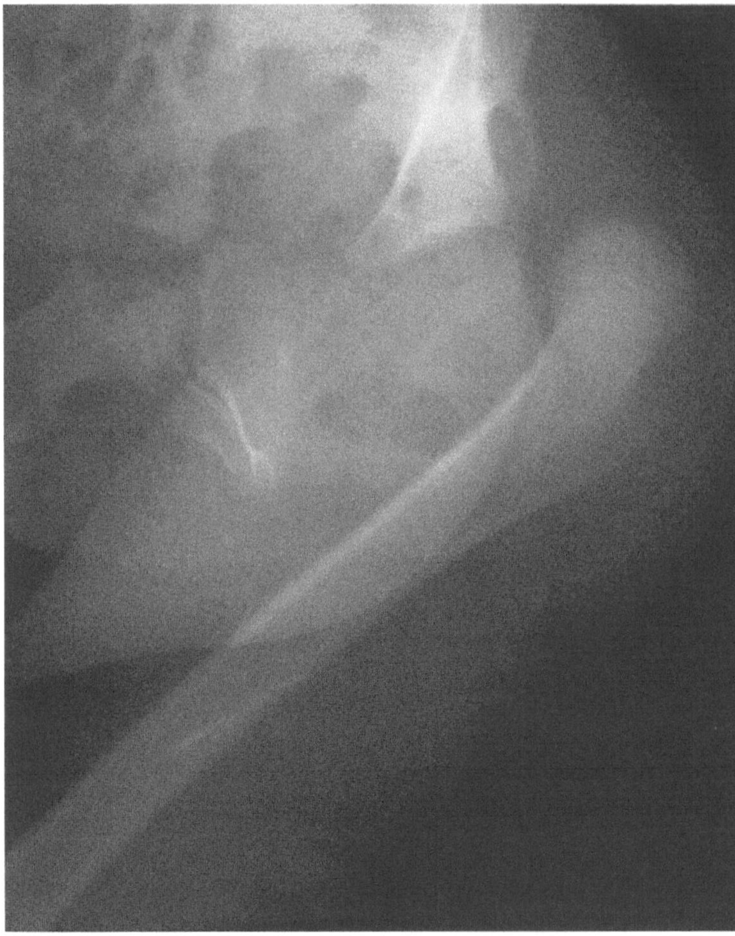

Fig. 4.3. Same case as in Fig. 4.2. True cross table view of the left hip clearly showing displacement of the femoral head posteriorly to the inhabited acetabulum. The dislocated hip underwent closed reduction within 6 h of the accident. One year later the child was free of symptoms and X-rays were normal

information about the exact topography of the fracture lines or of the displacement of the fragments in the sagital direction. The acetabular views of Judet et al. [249] are extremely useful in showing the fracture patterns of the acetabulum [20, 57, 91, 146, 351, 282, 388, 481, 497]. This is why all dislocated hips should be also assessed by these oblique acetabular views, in order to visualize associated fractures [87]. The internal oblique view or obturator view, which is taken with the patient supine and rotated through 45° away from the injured side, shows the full width of the obturator foramen, the iliopubic or anterior column, and the posterior acetabular lip (Fig. 4.4). The external oblique view, or ala view, is taken with the patient supine and rotated through 45° towards the injured hip and shows a flat frontal view of the iliac wing, the ilio-ischial or posterior column and the anterior lip of the acetabulum (Fig. 4.5).

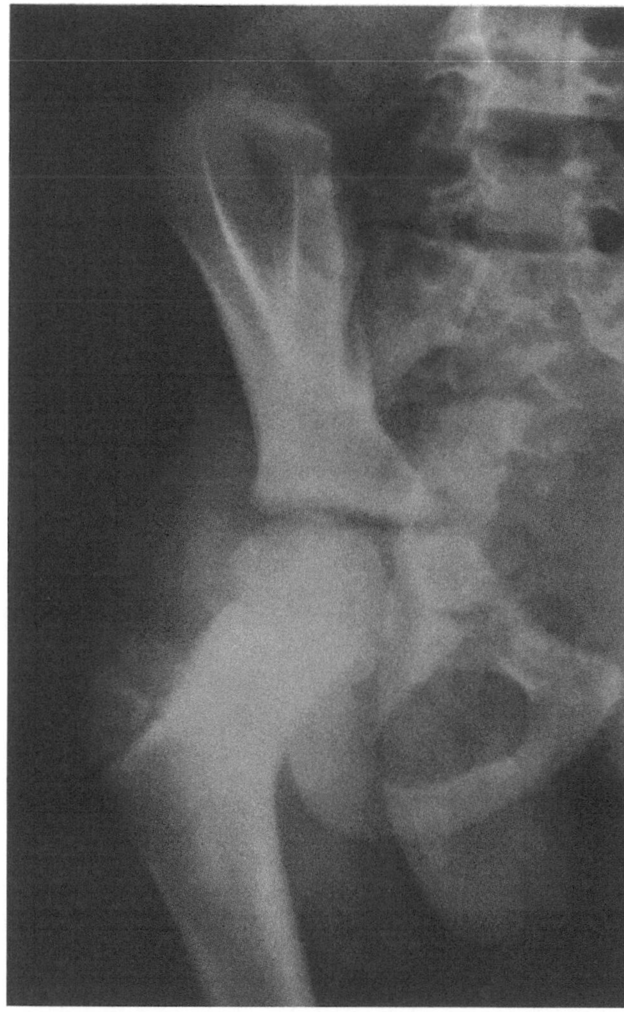

Fig. 4.4. Internal radiological oblique view or obturator view [249] of the acetabulum. The patient is supine and tilted 45° away from the injured side. Note the full width of the obturator foramen, the iliopubic or anterior column, and the posterior acetabular lip

The computerized axial tomographic (CAT) scan has been shown in the past few years to be extremely useful in defining the fracture pattern and the amount and type of displacement of fragments [30, 70, 481], as well as the operability of the acetabular fracture.

The roentgenographic diagnosis of the bone joint lesions in a child possibly presenting a THD must follow a protocol which should consist of standard views, i. e., frontal pelvic and true cross-table hip views, and Judet's special acetabular views. CAT scans should be added whenever diagnostic doubts or lack of information remains. This radiological protocol is also essential in those special circumstances

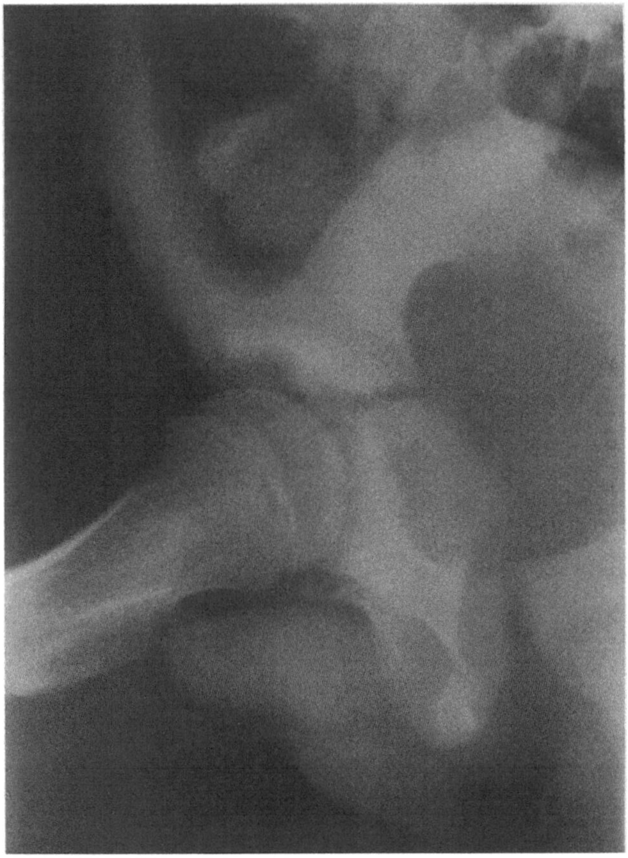

Fig. 4.5. External oblique view or ala view [249] of the acetabulum. The patient is supine and tilted 45° to the injured side. Note the flat frontal view of the iliac wing, the ilio-ischial or posterior column, and the anterior lip of the acetabulum

where there is a high risk of initially missing a THDC, i. e., a multiply-injured child or a child presenting a femoral shaft fracture, in order to definitely eliminate the occurrence of neglected THDC.

However, radiographic quality is often impaired in severely traumatized patients, due to the clinical restrictions imposed on X-ray examination [178]. These technically somewhat imperfect radiograms may result in the failure to detect acetabular fractures. Garvan recently reported a case of delayed presentation of posterior FD of the hip in a child [178]. The initial anteroposterior and lateral X-rays of the affected hip dislocation in Garvan's case appeared normal. Medical examination 6 weeks later revealed an old posterior FD of the hip, though no history of further injury to the patient was detected. Scott and Thomas suggested two possible explanations for this phenomenon of delayed presentation: (a) "acetabular fracture without dislocation was suffered at the time of injury," and the hip, being unstable, dislocated later on; and (b) "acetabular fracture with subluxation or dislocation was suffered, but the displacement was unwittingly reduced by the ambulance attendants either at the scene of the accident or during the journey to the hospital" [449]. Garvan's case provides additional documentation to demonstrate that the radiologic protocol described above should not only be technically "perfect" – as much as possible – but should also be subjected to careful scrutiny in order to avoid the diagnostic pitfalls of hip joint injuries [178].

4.3 Initial Therapeutic Protocol

4.3.1 Simple Dislocations

Hip dislocations should be immediately treated in order to prevent and minimize complications: gentle closed reduction under general anesthesia, with deep muscle relaxation, is to be attempted as soon as possible, preferably within 3–4 hours [19, 21, 29, 42, 74, 98, 103, 107, 113, 146, 168, 201, 211, 230, 236, 289, 322, 329, 332, 351, 356, 361, 383, 400, 411, 413, 438, 448]. Maneuvers should be performed with extreme gentleness in order to avoid further injuries to the bone joint and femoral head vessels [74, 103, 168, 169, 361, 411, 412, 448]. The importance of this careful manipulation in preventing a separation of the capital femoral epiphysis in a child has been previously emphasized [101, 141, 159, 351, 406]. Repeated attempts at closed reduction are particularly unadvisable.

Closed reduction of simple THDC under general anesthesia within hours of the accident is possible in most instances, and indeed achievable with ease [21, 68, 69, 74, 98, 144, 146, 163, 169, 211, 320, 326, 329, 361, 381, 406, 411, 412, 413, 424, 441].

However, it can be conceded that for extremely unusual cases with significant problems in anesthetic management, the reduction of a THDC may be gently performed with analgesia alone [325, 489].

4.3.1.1 Reduction Procedures

Several methods are currently used for closed reduction of THD, each group of authors giving preference to one of them. Some of these procedures are separately described for posterior and anterior dislocations, as follows.

Posterior Dislocations. The *Allis method* is the author's preferred procedure. This method restores the position of the head of the femur in a stepwise manner in the reverse order of displacement. The patient is placed supine on the floor and the pelvis is held by an assistant by firmly pressing on the anterior superior spines. The hip and knee are both flexed to 90°, with the thigh in its position of adduction and internal rotation. Flexion of the thigh relaxes the Y-ligament, an obstacle to reduction of regular dislocations. Traction directly upwards, with both hands of the operator behind the knee, will lift the femoral head over the acetabular rim, through the capsular rent, into the acetabular cavity. Abduction and external rotation may be useful in the last step of the procedure. The leg will be extended after the head is inside the acetabulum and only then; no effort of extension should be made before reduction of the dislocation, as leverage against the acetabulum may produce further joint injuries. A palpable and audible "clunk" [63] usually occurs when the dislocation is reduced, but this is not absolute. Very little force should be applied because the Allis procedure aims to avoid further laceration of the joint structures [467].

The *Stimson method* aims at reduction following the same general principle as Allis, but places the patient prone on a table, with both lower limbs hanging over the end of the table. An assistant presses the sacrum, and the surgeon flexes the knee at a right angel, and applies firm downward pressure on the lower leg until reduction is accomplished.

In the *Bigelow method* the initial steps of the procedure are similar to those of Allis: patient supine on the floor, countertraction applied to anterior superior iliac spines by an assistant, and hip and knee both flexed at 90°. Then, the thigh is gently rotated internally and externally, and also rocked forward and backward, to disengage the head from the muscles and the posterior capsule. Reduction is accomplished by further external rotation and abduction of the thigh.

The method of Allis is preferable to that of Bigelow, which is considered somewhat hazardous. According to Allis, "methods of restoration by means of rotation and circumduction are unphilosophical because they do not compel the head to return by its way of exit, and dangerous because they enlarge the torn area and have an unfavourable tendency to force capsule and other foreign material into the socket" [5]. Although the Stimson method is safe and effective, it requires a prone position, which is frequently unadvisable in multiply-injured patients, and it may provide difficulties in determining the clinical stability of the hip [382].

Anterior Dislocations. The *Allis method* is extremely useful in achieving closed reduction of obturator dislocations. The patient is placed supine on the floor, the pelvis is held down by an assistant and traction is applied to the thigh in upward direction. While traction is maintained, the thigh is gently adducted and intrarotated, which helps in bringing the head into the acetabulum. Then, the leg is extended to the floor. As stated by Speed, too much flexion must be avoided, as it pushes the head farther into the obturator depression [467]. Slight forward traction is the force needed to lift the head near the capsular rent.

This procedure, however, is inappropriate for pubic dislocations because it tightens the already taut posterior capsular structures of the hip, which bind the head firmly on the pubis [87, 122]. The first step toward achieving reduction of a pubic dislocation is hyperextension of the hip, as described by *Dingley and Denham* [122]. The patient is placed supine on a table, and countertraction is applied to the anterior superior iliac spines. The lower limbs are left hanging over the table edge and the hip is hyperextended, while traction is applied along the axis of the femur. Gentle intrarotation of the femur will then lead to reduction of the dislocation, aided by an assistant who places direct downward pressure over the femoral head [87, 122].

Inferior Dislocations. Closed reduction of luxatio erecta is achieved by traction in a cephalad direction, along the axis of the femur, together with countertraction by holding down the pelvis, which is performed by an assistant. A mild internal rotation [2, 407, 437], or possibly extrarotation, may have to be added in certain instances. Extension of the limb should not be performed until the femoral head is seated in the acetabular socket.

4.3.1.2 Postreduction Clinical and Radiological Tests

Clinical Test of Stable Reduction. The stability of reduction must be immediately tested after maneuvers have been performed; to obtain the best efficiency for this test, the general anesthesia and muscle relaxation must still be deep. The hip joint must be stable in a full range of motion, which must be explored carefully.

Radiological Diagnosis of Full Reduction. Even when reduction appears stable enough through clinical tests, the child should remain anesthetized, as a radiological examination is the definitive means of diagnosing complete reduction. An anteroposterior view of the pelvis and lateral views of both hips are essential to permit comparison of the "reduced" hip with the uninvolved one. A careful inspection of Shenton's line and of the comparative dimensions of the femoral heads are useful as guidelines indicating a disturbed hip. A basic sign of reduction is to find the femoral head concentrically centered into the acetabulum However, the essential sign of full reduction is the width of the medial joint space of the hip, which must be identical to that of the contralateral hip (Fig. 4.6).

Radiological Diagnosis of Joint Fractures Possibly Initially Overlooked. Sometimes acetabular or proximal femoral fractures, missed in prereduction radiograms, become evident after reduction [197, 351], diagnosis changing from simple dislocation to FD. Further management of this condition will be analyzed later on.

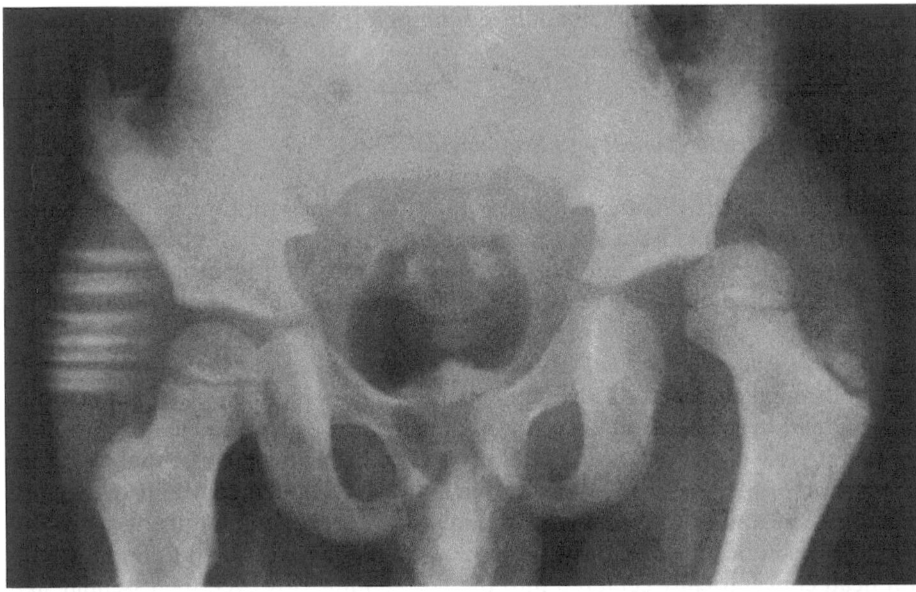

a

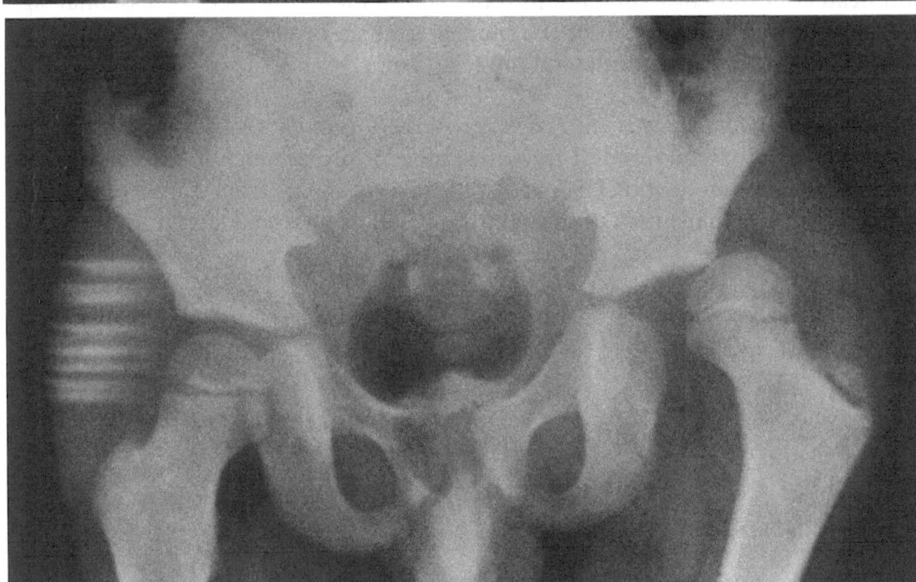

b

Fig. 4.6 a–c. Posterior dislocation of left hip in a 7-year-old girl who fell while running. **a** At admission. **b** Frontal radiogram showing full reduction: the medial joint space is identical in both hips. A true cross-table radiogram confirmed diagnosis of complete reduction. Closed reduction was achieved within 6 h of the accident, and skin traction was applied for 4 weeks. **c** Ten years later there is normal morphology of the left hip and full function

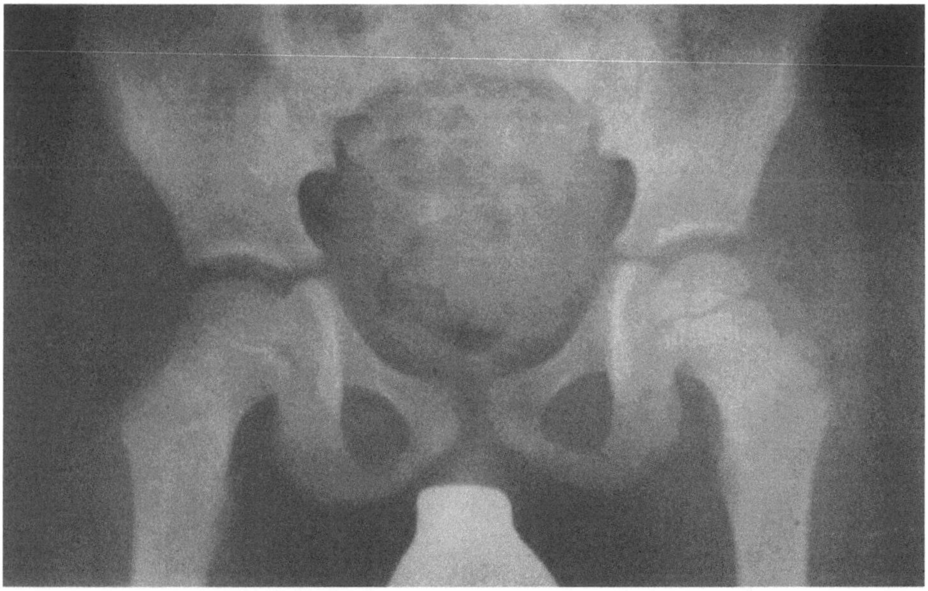

c

4.3.1.3 Irreducible Recent Simple Dislocations

Failure of early closed reduction maneuvers in simple THDC is uncommon [19, 21, 101, 103, 166, 339]. The reported incidence of these irreducible recent simple dislocations in children has ranged between 2.5% and 16% [70, 146, 172, 348, 366], and I found it in 6% of a 38-case series collected in Uruguay. While reviewing the WS, 39 such cases were found [21, 22, 63, 69, 70, 78, 95, 146, 155, 166, 172, 176, 244, 332, 339, 348, 366, 385, 429, 435, 465, 482, 519]. Thirty-three of these cases had been operated upon and their pathoanatomical bases are known.

Concerning the anatomoclinical features of this entity, the cases seem to fall naturally in two types [22, 72]: *nonreduced dislocations,* with closed maneuvers under general anesthesia being clearly unsuccessful, which is confirmed by the radiological image of a persistent dislocated hip in the post-maneuvers control (Fig. 4.7); and *nonconcentric reductions,* with apparent clinical achievement of closed reduction, but with the postmaneuvers radiogram showing that the femoral head is not fully reduced, i. e., medial diastasis between head and socket, with respect to the contralateral hip joint (Fig. 4.8) [22, 63, 70, 72, 146, 166, 201, 332, 348, 385, 413].

Pathoanatomical Basis. Irreducible recent simple dislocations are the result of soft tissue interposition between the femoral head and the acetabulum. Several anatomical structures may prevent closed reduction in these cases, i. e., the joint capsule, the acetabular labrum, the periarticular muscles, cartilaginous loose bodies, and less frequently, the ligamentum teres and the acetabular edge. Each of these structures may be the only interposed soft tissue, or may be associated with some other soft tissue.

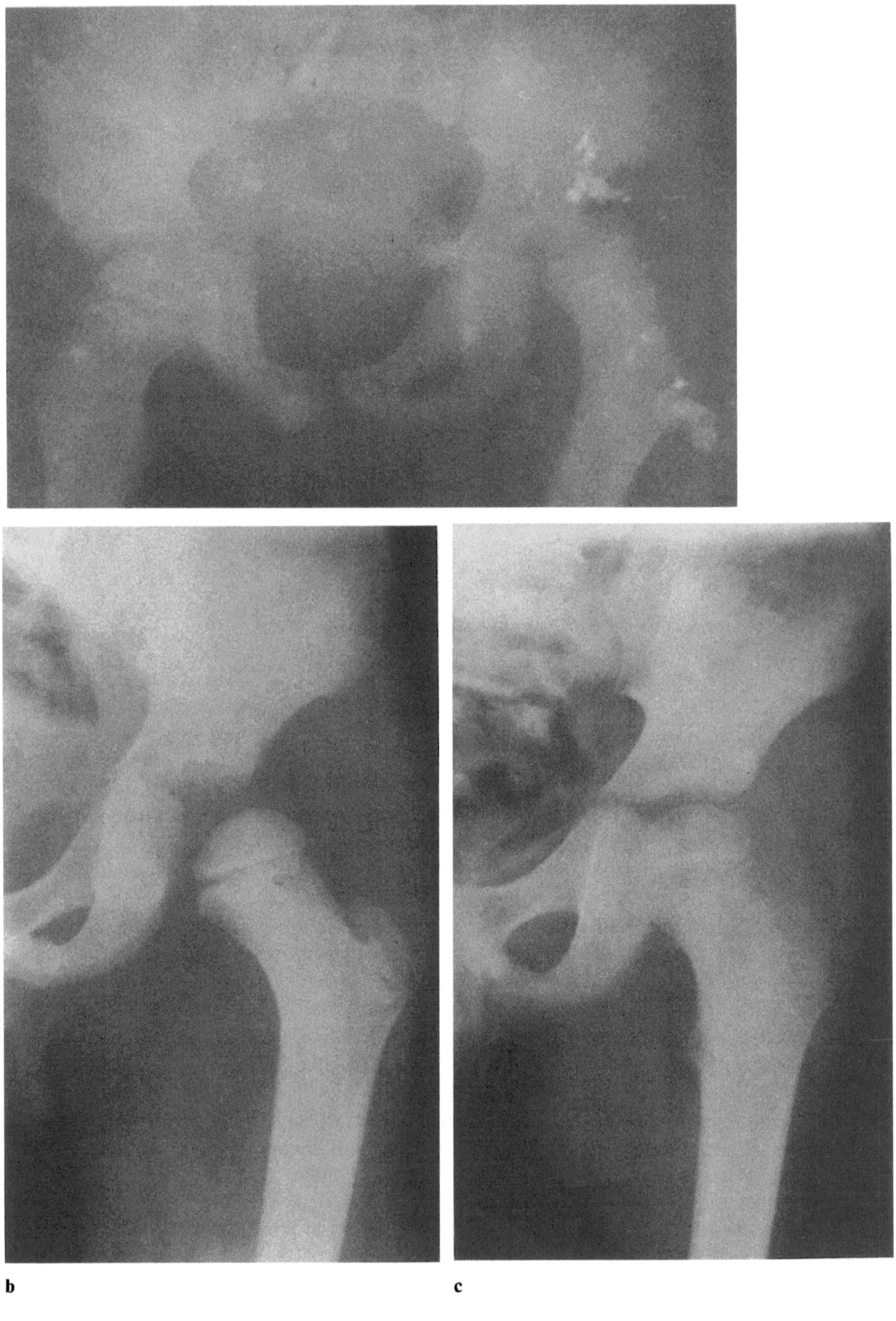

a

b

c

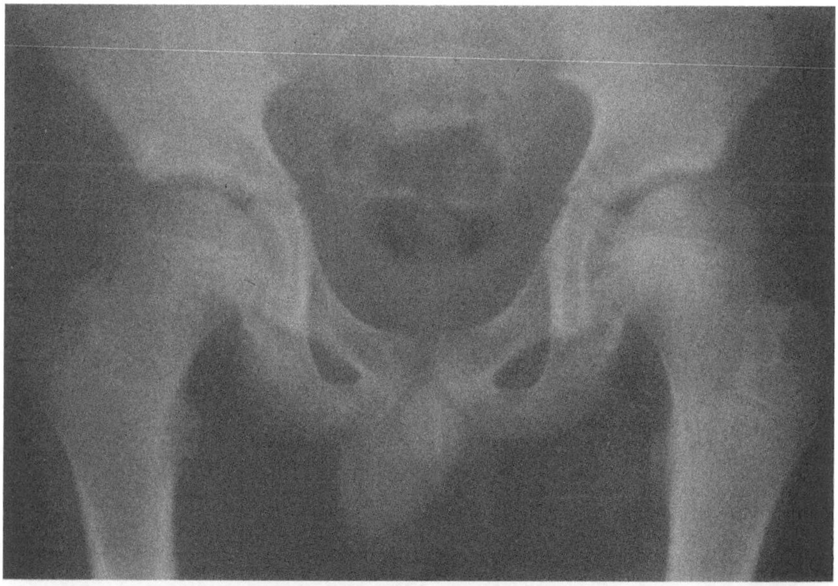
d

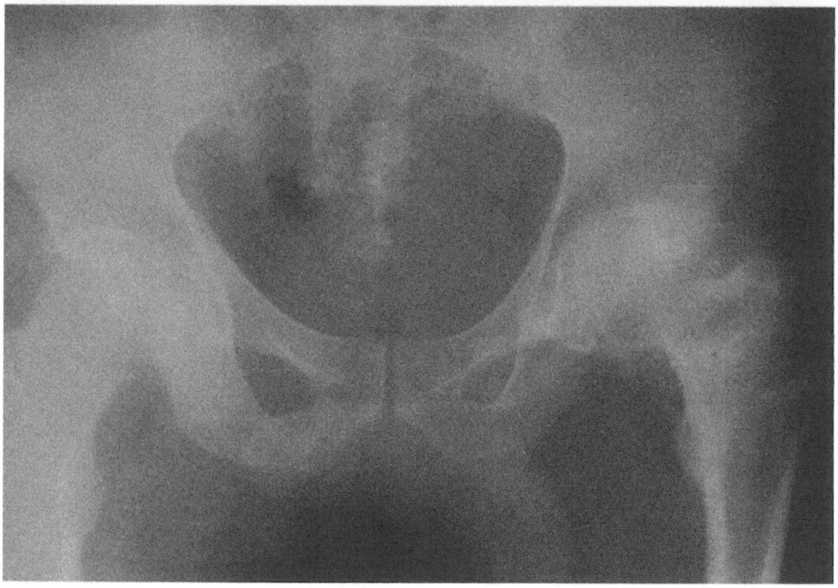
e

Fig. 4.7 a–e. Nonreduction dislocation after attempt at closed reduction. **a** Posterior dislocation of the left hip in a 7-year-old boy, following a fall while playing football. **b** Radiogram after closed maneuvers: the femoral head, though in front of the acetabulum, is clearly nonreduced. **c** Following open reduction 3 days later, with pulling of a detached portion of the acetabular labrum and a capsular flap out of the socket. The femoral head is fully reduced into the acetabulum; **d** Condition 6 years later: diffuse damage to the growth plate, predominating at its lateral side, has occurred. Asymmetrical widening and shortening of the femoral neck has led to valgus angulation. The femoral head has grown in accordance with its modified base, and coxa magna has resulted. **e** Thirty years later there is severe traumatic arthritis, with significant functional limitation and further treatment being planned. (Fig. 4.7 b, reprinted from Barquet [22], and Fig. 4.7 d reprinted from Barquet [27])

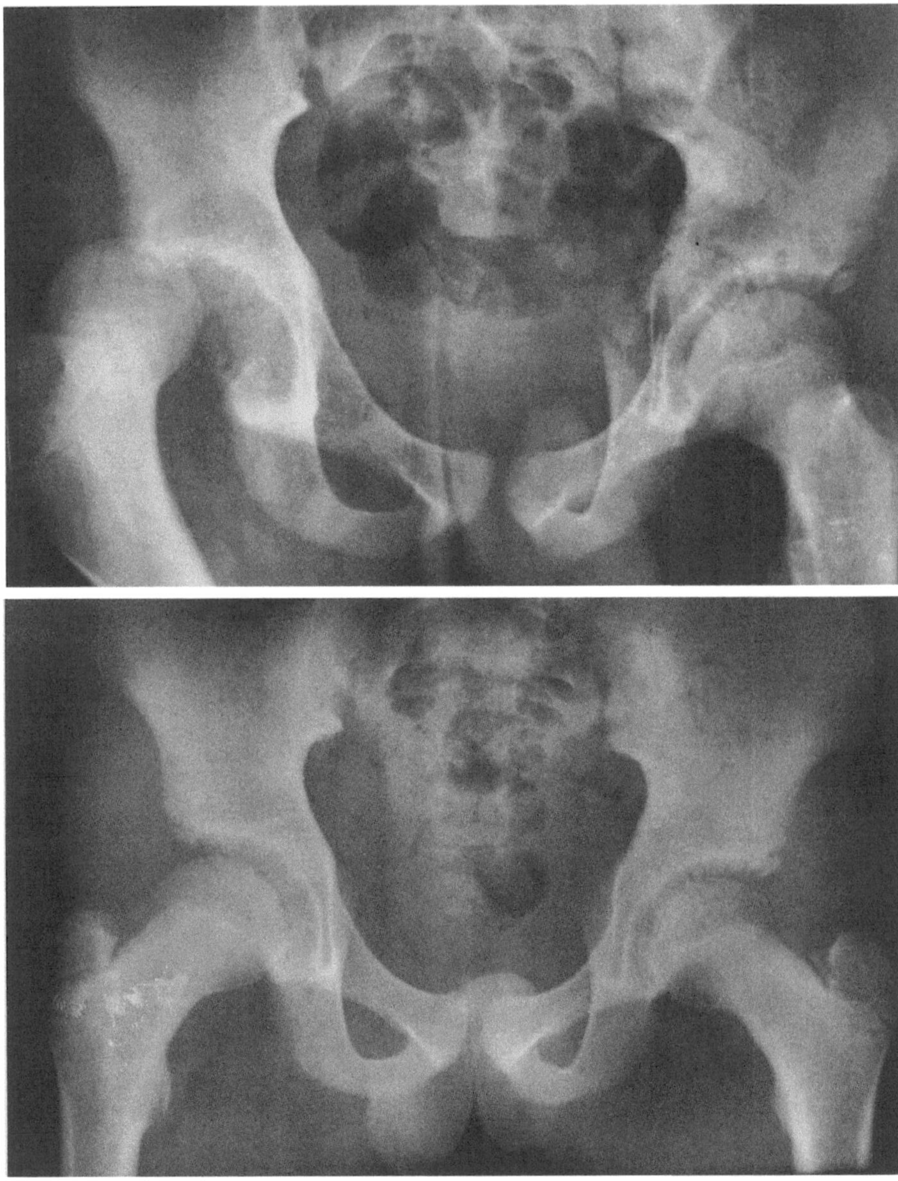

a

b

Fig. 4.8 a, b. Nonconcentric reduction after closed maneuvers. **a** Posterior dislocation of the right hip in a 13-year-old boy, following a traffic accident. **b** Condition after closed maneuvers: although Shenton's line seems normal and the dimensions of the femoral head appear identical to those of the contralateral head, the medial joint space of the right hip is greater than that of the left hip

Infolding or invagination of a flap of the torn *capsule* into the joint, as a result of closed maneuvers, provides an obstacle to reduction of the dislocation. Funk reported the interposition of a capsular flap preventing reduction [172], and others have described the associated infolding of the torn capsule and other soft structures [22, 63]. Buttonholing of the femoral head through a capsular tear leads to entrapment of head, rendering closed manipulations inefficient [70, 146, 176, 366]. Nerubay found an anterior dislocation with a buttonhole tear of the anterior capsule and interposition of muscles [339].

In posterior dislocations, the *acetabular labrum* is sometimes partially detached from the acetabulum by the displaced femoral head, as a "bucket handle" tear in a knee meniscus [110]. If the torn labrum is introduced into the joint by the femoral head during attempts to replace it, complete reduction may be blocked [110, 166, 364, 464]. Interposition of the labrum in THDC has been found by itself [22, 70, 78, 146, 348, 465] and in association with other soft tissue structures [22, 63, 70, 166].

Periarticular muscles may also be involved as interposed structures, rendering closed reduction impossible. The pathoanatomy of irreducibility of muscular origin is similar to that of capsular origin, i. e., interposition of a muscular flap or tendon, or buttonholing of the femoral head through a muscular tear. Campbell found interposition of the tendinous aponeurosis and insertion of the external rotators [69], while Wilson described the short external rotators as torn and sucked into the acetabulum [519]. In Nebrubay's case the interposed muscles were the rectus femoris and the iliopsoas tendon [339]. Buttonholing of the femoral head through a psoas muscle tear has also been reported [155].

Ligamentum teres interposition [332, 482] and *curling of the acetabular edge* [435, 482] are less frequent causes of irreducible recent pediatric TDH. Interposition of *cartilaginous loose bodies* – or osteocartilaginous loose fragments, usually invisible with X-rays – resulting from tangential trauma to the articular surface of the acetabulum or femoral head and preventing reduction has been described in recent simple THDC, isolated or in association with other soft tissues [63, 70, 146, 166, 185, 244].

Diagnosis. The definite diagnosis of irreducible THD is radiological, as stated above. An arthrogram might be performed, but in the acutely luxated hip, extravasation of the dye through the capsular tear would make interpretation of this examination difficult [351]. A CAT scan would also be useful [30, 70, 351]. However, a careful scrutiny of anteroposterior and lateral radiological views after closed maneuvers seems sufficient to disclose whether or not a THD has been fully reduced.

Treatment. Repeated closed attempts are contraindicant [22, 146, 460]. Immediate open reduction is to be performed in order to remove the obstacle and achieve full reduction: if an incongruous reduction persists due to an interposed soft tissue structure, damage to the joint will occur, possibly leading to traumatic arthritis [70, 72].

The surgical approach will depend on the variety of dislocation: posterior approach in posterior dislocation, and anterior approach in anterior luxation.

Nonreduced dislocations permit a wide inspection of the interposed structures, but in the case of nonconcentric reduction the femoral head should be redislocated to adequately assess the hip joint and the anatomic structures preventing full reduction. When buttonholing has occurred, the opening in the capsule or muscle should be extended to reduce the luxation. If interposition of a tendinomuscular structure is present, this should be retracted and the pathway of the head freed: the tendon might be cut if it definitely interferes with reduction, and immediately repaired. In nonconcentric reduction, the capsular tear should be enlarged to free the femoral head. When a "bucket handle" tear of the labrum is interposed, the detached portion of the labrum should be pulled out of the socket, the dislocation reduced, and the labrum reinserted or repaired if possible, or eventually excised. When a capsular flap is inverted, it should be pulled out of the socket. Loose cartilaginous bodies should be removed after redislocation, and the capsule should be carefully repaired after full reduction has been achieved.

Intraoperative anteroposterior and lateral radiographical views should be routinely performed to confirm that full reduction has been surgically achieved.

4.3.2 Fracture Dislocations

4.3.2.1 Dislocations with Acetabular Fracture

Posterior Type 1 FD. A therapeutic protocol similar to that for simple dislocations is advocated in those posterior dislocations with minor acetabular fractures, i.e., stable type after reduction [70, 146, 400]. As for simple dislocations, reduction and stability after closed maneuvers should be evaluated by clinical and radiological procedures, as described above. Frontal, lateral, and oblique roentgenographic views are necessary to evaluate concentric reduction of the dislocation and the definitive position of the small acetabular fragment.

Irreducible recent posterior type 1 FD are also uncommon, and may be the result of soft tissue interposition, as in simple dislocations, though more frequently a small osseous or osteocartilaginous fragment blocks reduction. Open reduction is obviously necessary in these cases.

Posterior FD Types 2, 3, and 4. Some authors favor an initial closed reduction of these FD, followed by reassessment of the fracture pattern and stability of the joint. They advise open procedures only when closed reduction fails, when loose fragments are visible in the joint space on roentgenograms, and when reduction is unstable [57, 70, 81, 400, 473, 517].

However, there is significant data supporting the view that these complex injuries should be treated by primary open procedures, both in children and in adults [8, 107, 146, 486, 500]. Epstein argues that closed reduction is not to be attempted, and bone and cartilage fragments must be surgically removed before the dislocation is reduced [146]. The loose fragments, which are found in the hip joint in a high percentage of cases, would be responsible for incongruity of the joint surfaces and for a greater tendency toward disintergration of the joint [146, 500]. The removal of these loose bodies from the acetabular socket would diminish the incidence of traumatic arthritis and, together with restoration of the acetabulum by surgical reduction and internal fixation of the acetabular fracture, would be the procedure of choice in the management of these serious injuries, as found by several authors [8, 107, 146, 383, 410a, 486, 500]. For children with life-threatening injuries, when the general condition contraindicates a major operation of the hip initially, early closed reduction of the dislocation is to be accepted; a delay of few days before removing loose fragments from the joint space and the stabilization of the "unstable" hip joint is better than nothing in these instances [256].

The value of the CAT scan in adequately disclosing the exact type of fragments and displacement must be emphasized in these FD. This information will help in planning the open procedure.

The large acetabular fragments should be internally fixed with Kirschner wires in young children (under 10 or 11 years of age), and the wires removed when sufficient healing provides stability. For older children, screws and possibly plates may be used [107]. Whichever the chosen implant, it must not damage the triradiate acetabular cartilage [351], especially in younger children, in order to prevent further serious consequences in the development of the acetabulum.

The Kocher-Gibson approach should be used for these posterior FD. The large fragment, responsible for instability, must be managed with extreme care, preserving its soft tissue connections [191], and repositioned looking for anatomic reduction. A mini towel clip is useful to achieve this reduction, which will be transitorily fixed with Kirschner wires. Radiological views will help in assessing the correct reduction of the bone fragment and position of the wires, which will be either definitely left in place, changed to a new site, or replaced by screws or plates, according to the age of the child and special conditions of the injury (Figs. 4.9 and 4.10).

Anterior FD. These are exceptional injuries, and their therapeutic protocol should be guided by the same principles as posterior FD.

4.3.2.2 Dislocations with Femoral Head Fracture

There is no general agreement concerning the management of this injury, as a result of its extreme rarity.

Posterior dislocations with shear fractures of the femoral head in children are very difficult to treat. However, an important trend of opinion recommending primary open procedures for this complex lesion in adults [84, 146, 284, 422] may be applied to children. Thorough debridement and removal of all small cartilaginous fragments which may become abrasive agents is a main part of this therapeutic protocol. Roeder and DeLee recommend restoring the hip joint surfaces to as congruous a state as possible [422]. This especially applies to Pipkin type 2 FD: reduction and fixation of the fragment to the remainder of the femoral head by pins or screws, and reduction of the dislocation appears an ideal solution. However, this is a very difficult task. Pipkin type 1 lesions may well be treated by the primary open procedure, although it involves the removal of the caudad fragment, which is usually too small and does not belong to the weight-bearing site. Prognosis is guarded in these FD, since avascular necrosis and traumatic arthritis are extremely frequent, and results are fair or poor. Nevertheless, a careful primary open procedure has been suggested as the only way of enhance this poor prognosis.

a

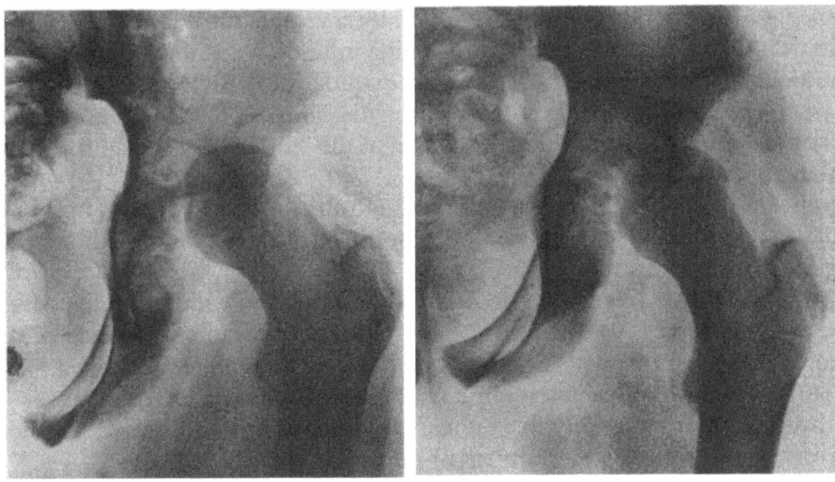

b

c

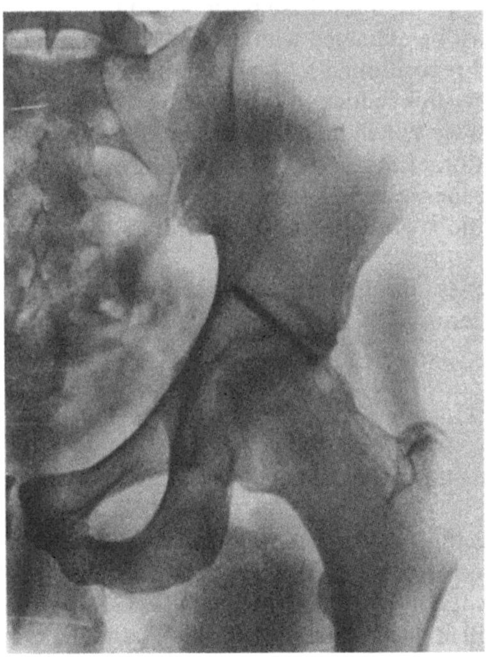

Fig. 4.9. a Posterior dislocation of the left hip with fracture of the posterior rim and wall in a 13-year-old boy following a traffic accident. Closed reduction of the dislocation and spica cast applied for 1 month. **b** Redislocation 3 months later. Immediate reduction of the luxation and internal fixation of the acetabular fragment with a screw performed 15 days later. Nonreduction and nonfixation of the acetabular fragment at the time of injury were the cause of instability. **c** Perfect clinical and radiological result 13 years later. (From Rigault et al. [413])

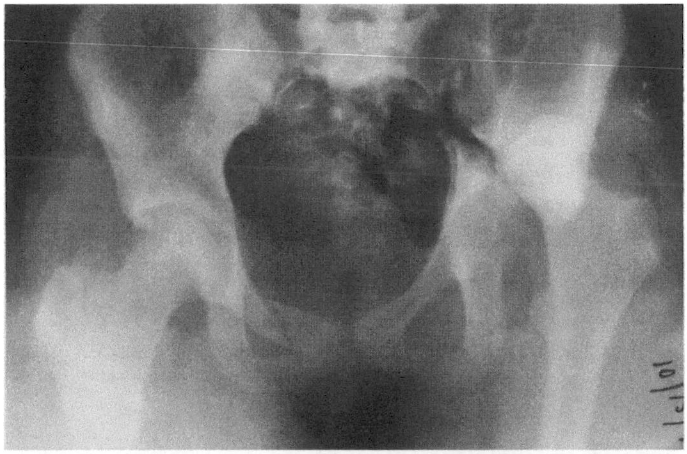

a

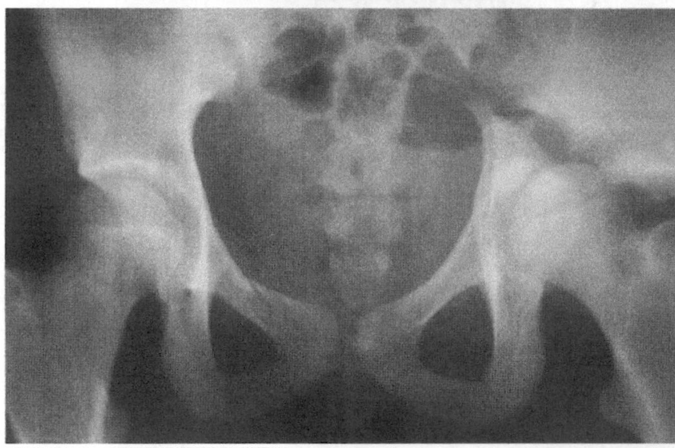

b

c

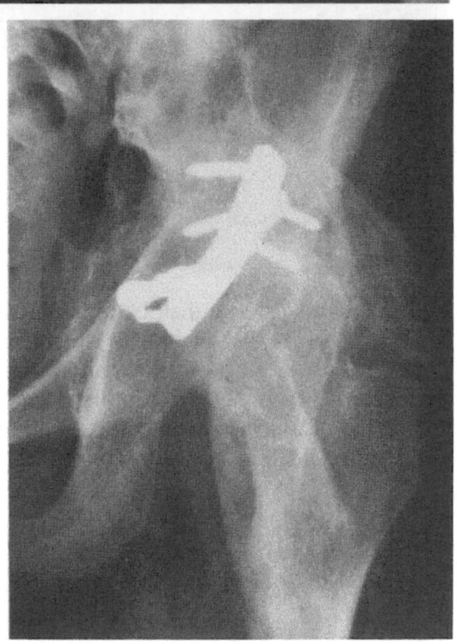

Fig. 4.10 a–c. Girl (14 year old) injured her left hip in an automobile accident. **a** After accident: posterior dislocation with anterior and posterior acetabular fracture with comminution. **b** Closed reduction within 12 h of the accident. Three days later open reduction and internal fixation of the acetabulum with a plate. **c** Condition 5 months later: extra-articular heterotopic bone and spontaneous intra-articular and extra-articular arthrodesis. (From Robertson and Peterson [420])

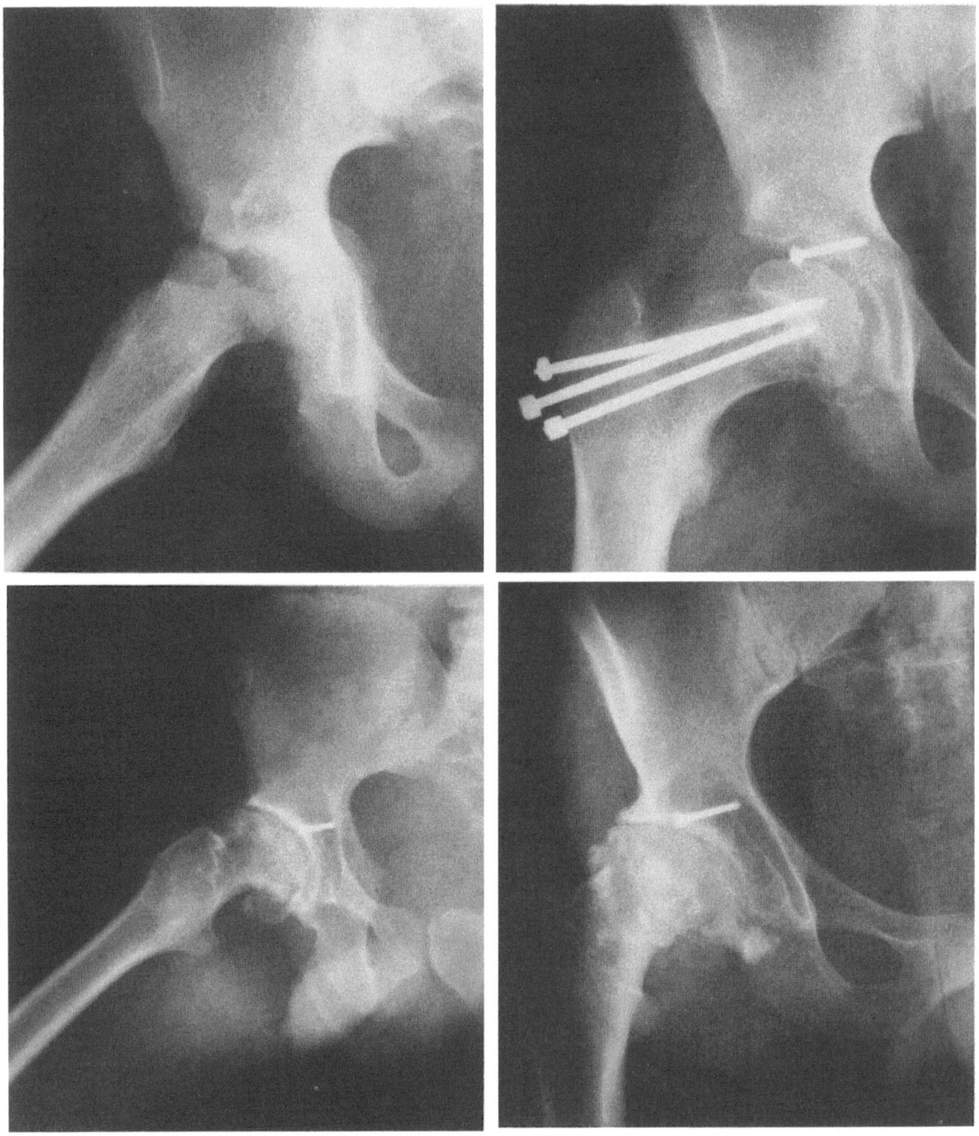

a b c d

Fig. 4.11 a–d. Posterior dislocation of hip and epiphyseal separation, and large posterior acetabular fracture in an 11-year-old boy. **a** At admission. Open reduction and fixation of the epiphyseal separation with three Knowles pins, and fixation of posterior acetabular fragment with one screw was performed 11 days later. **b** Condition 3 months after reduction. The proximal femoral extremity developed avascular necrosis. **c** and **d** Eighteen years later, joint line, though preserved, is narrowed, and femoral head is flattened (coxa plana). (From Fina and Kelly [160])

Anterior dislocations with compression fractures of the femoral head are to be initially treated as simple dislocations. However, the evolution of these lesions should be periodically controlled because the development of segmental avascular necrosis in the compressed area is highly likely [236]. Whenever this complication develops, precocious reconstructive surgery to the hip should be performed; intertrochanteric osteotomies would, by changing the weight-bearing site of the femoral head, prevent further collapse in this necrotic area, and a better outcome may be achieved [236] (Fig. 3.14).

4.3.2.3 Dislocations with Separation of the Capital Femoral Epiphysis

Prognosis for hip dislocations with separation of the capital epiphysis of the femur (HDSCFE) type 1 is far less favorable than for other types of FD of the hip. Avascular necrosis seems inevitable, regardless of the interval before reduction and the reduction-fixation procedure.

Although removal of the dislocated separated epiphysis has been applied [67, 440], there is general agreement nowadays on the use of a reconstructive protocol. Closed reduction in these cases is obviously inefficient. Open reduction is to be performed using a posterolateral approach, which facilitates reduction and internal fixation of the epiphysis to the femoral neck, and repositioning of the epiphysis into the acetabulum. For internal fixation, two or three Kirschner wires should be used [31, 55, 271, 310, 427, 514], in order to protect the physis from the additional damage produced by threaded implants, especially in young children [31, 310]. A spica cast must supplement fixation during a 6- to 8-week period.

Provided early anatomical reduction and fixation is performed, prognosis for HDSCFE type 2 appears better, as the remaining blood supply to the epiphysis is larger [310]. This lesion requires open and precocious reduction of the proximal femoral unit, with accurate protection against further separation of the capital epiphysis. Fixation with Kirschner wires supplemented with cast immobilization is essential.

This active therapeutic protocol for HDSCFE types 1 and 2 has permitted the achievement of fair results in certain instances, a gratifying outcome considering the obvious poor prognosis of this injury (Figs. 3.16 and 4.11)! This protocol is also recommended because it preserves bone tissue, which would be necessary for secondary reconstructive surgical procedures, such as arthrodesis and arthroplasty, a possibility that must be anticipated in every patient with this complex injury.

4.3.2.4 Dislocations with Femoral Neck Fracture

Since this injury and its prognosis are so similar to HDSCFE, the therapeutic principles should also be the same, i. e., surgical anatomical reduction and fixation as an emergency approach.

A posterolateral approach is used. The FD is carefully exposed and capsulotomy is completed. The femoral neck fracture is anatomically reduced and temporarily fixed with Kirschner wires entering through the lateral trochanteric cortex and traversing the fracture site [53]. The femoral head is then repositioned into the acetabular socket with extreme care. Definitive fixation of the fracture is carried out with two cancellous screws, preferably of the small fragment ASIF set, taking extreme care not to damage the epiphyseal growth plate [53, 216, 333, 379, 408]. This plate should not be traversed by the screws. These implants permit one to achieve stable fixation through interfragmentary compression.

A spica cast should be applied to maintain the dislocated hip joint immobilized. The immobilization period will be discussed in Chap. 5.

As also stated for HDSCFE, early reduction and internal fixation in dislocations with femoral neck fracture will probably not prevent the development of avascular necrosis, but will make any further reconstructive surgery easier (Fig. 3.18).

4.3.2.5 Dislocations with Separation of the Greater Trochanter

Partial avulsions of the greater trochanter should be immobilized in abduction and slight external rotation for 6 weeks, usually in a one and one-half spica cast.

A completely avulsed trochanter is an indication for surgery. The trochanter should be reduced by open procedures [31, 91, 107, 351], some smooth Kirschner wires inserted proximally, anchored in the proximal shaft distally, and secured with a tension band wire looped over them [333, 511]. This procedure provides stability and interferes less with future trochanteric growth (Fig. 3.19). Once sound healing has been achieved, the implants are to be removed.

Prognosis in this FD is guarded, as growth disturbances may follow, as will be analyzed in Chap. 5.

4.3.3 Dislocations with Ipsilateral Femoral Shaft Fracture

In this combined injury, closed reduction of the dislocated hip by simple manipulation has been considered not only difficult, as the long lever of the femoral shaft cannot be used, but also dangerous because it might involve further damage to the soft tissues at the femoral fracture site [139, 218]. However, Connolly has found that occasionally with distal femoral fractures, closed reduction of the hip dislocation is possible by simple manipulation [87], and Gregory has stated that the point is to gain control of the proximal femoral fragment: "a straight manipulation seeking reduction may be tried, and occasionally it is successful" [191]. I was surprised to find, in the reviewed cases in the WS in which this associated injury had been treated early, that those precocious attempts at closed reduction by manipulation of the proximal shaft fragment, associated in some instances with pressing of the greater trochanter in posterior dislocations and of the femoral head in anterior dislocations, had been efficient in most instances, and no iatrogenic lesions were described in the clinical follow-up control [25]. This procedure applies when a long proximal femoral fragment exists, i.e., in mid and distal third shaft fractures, and such an attempt may be recommended.

If such an attempt fails or if the shaft fracture is proximal, certain other methods of "closed" reduction of the dislocation, which aim to indirectly manipulate the proximal femoral fragment via pins or screws fixed to the bone and connected to handling devices, are to be performed. Several such procedures have been recommended, using fixtures to either the greater trochanter or the femoral neck [51, 114, 213, 218, 235, 296, 307, 463, 520]. I prefer to use a tube or rod, attached with clamps or ball joints to two or three Schanz screws (ASIF or Hoffmann external fixation systems) inserted into the lateral aspect of the proximal shaft fragment (Fig. 4.12).

Approach to the shaft fracture site and purchase on the distal end of the proximal femoral fragment [218, 517] is to be performed only as a third line procedure, and situations requiring its use are extremely infrequent. Open reduction of the dislocation is to be used when previous methods have failed.

This protocol refers solely to simple dislocations and to those FD to be treated by closed procedures, i. e., type 1 FD, because other types of FD of the hip are to be treated by primary open procedures. The femoral shaft fracture in children is usually treated nonoperatively (traction and cast), a procedure which is most efficient in almost all instances.

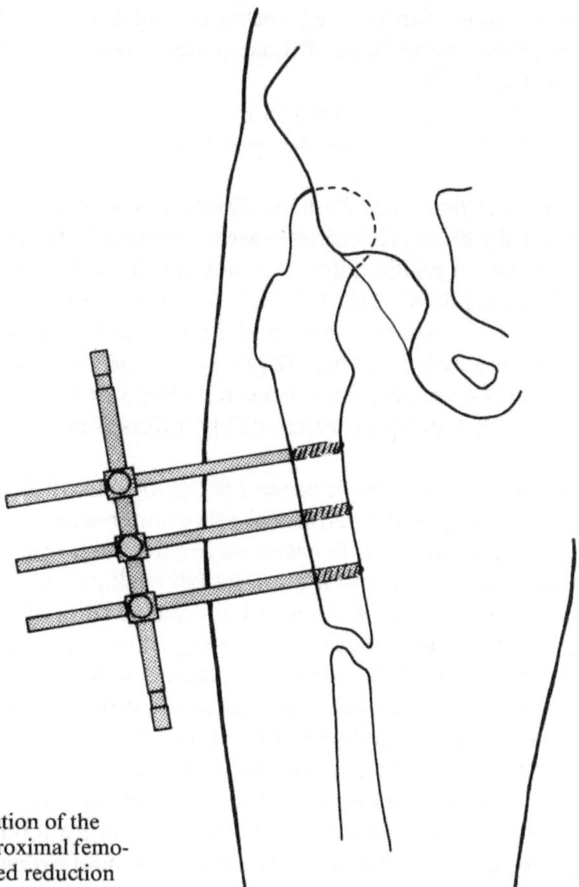

Fig. 4.12. Model showing the application of the ASIF external fixator to control the proximal femoral fragment, in order to achieve closed reduction of a hip dislocation associated with a concomitant ipsilateral femoral shaft fracture.

4.3.4 Dislocations with Nerve Injuries

There are several possible outcomes in nerve injuries associated with THDC: (a) a total sciatic palsy may show early and complete recovery (neurapraxia of the nerve), or a permanent or prolonged deficiency of peroneal nerve function and complete recovery of the tibial nerve, indicating stretching of the nerve root, with neurapraxia of S1 and neurotmesis or axonotmesis of L4 and L5; and (b) an isolated peroneal nerve deficiency may show two different outcomes: either rapid complete recovery, indicating neurapraxia of the peripheral nerve or of the L5 nerve root, or a persistent or prolonged (6–24 months) deficiency, occurring in neurotmesis or axonotmesis of the L5 nerve root [112, 382, 485].

Previous authors have considered that the neurologic deficiency in THDC shows a higher degree of regression than in adults [101, 413]. However, this has not been confirmed while reviewing the WS. However, it is interesting to note, as Seddon has emphasized, that there is a lack of correlation between neurological and functional recovery with respect to the sciatic nerve, with much better total function than anticipated by neurological examination. A protective sensation and acceptable walking function, except for having to wear a toe-rising device, may occur in a significant percentage of those patients without complete recovery of neurological function [450].

The therapeutic protocol in the case of associated nerve injuries to the THDC should thus be planned on these bases.

Sciatic Deficiency in Posterior Simple Dislocations. A sciatic palsy in a posterior simple dislocation is a further reason for immediate reduction. In posterior simple dislocations, a sciatic palsy does not appear to be an indication for early surgical exploration [20, 87, 112, 146, 382, 400, 500], because if nerve stretching has occurred, recovery is most probable, and if nerve root injury is the anatomical basis of the lesion, surgery is of no benefit [20, 87, 112, 382, 485]. However, certain authors consider that if no recovery has occurred after 3 or 4 weeks, the nerve should be explored [382, 400], a position which widely differs from that of Decoulx et al. [112].

Sciatic Deficiency in Posterior FD. Sciatic palsy in FD is more frequently dependent on stretching of the peripheral nerve or nerve root by the posteriorly dislocated femoral head. However, in case a large acetabular fragment, with or without comminution, is displaced, and it does not fall back into place after reduction of the dislocation, early open reduction and internal fixation of the fragment is necessary, which also permits exploration and freeing of the nerve in cases when it is being pressed upon [87, 400, 517], or repairing the nerve if it is lacerated. Therefore, the decision for nerve exploration in these instances is often aided by the fact that this operation would be indicated by fracture alone [281].

In posterior FD, sciatic deficiency or irritation may also be caused by progressive compression due to callus formation in cases where persistent displaced acetabular fragments are present. This is an indication for surgical decompression and excision of the offending bone fragments and callus [87, 191].

Femoral and Obturator Nerve Deficiency in Anterior Simple Dislocations. These injuries are dependent on stretching of these nerves and should be managed in a nonoperative regimen.

Rehabilitation Program – Palliative Surgery. A rehabilitation program should be instituted in order to maintain the lower limb in the best possible condition throughout the period of neurological deficiency. The limb is rehabilitated, with the skin and prevention of contractures being taken into consideration, and the appropriate splintage is applied to allow walking [256].

Palliative surgery may by necessary on bone joints and muscles in due time, when residual neurological damage is unavoidable. Tendon transfer or stabilization of the foot and ankle are commonly required in cases of permanent damage to the peroneal nerve.

4.3.5 Dislocations with Vascular Injuries

THDC must be urgently reduced in every case, but when signs of vascular compromise are present in anterior dislocations the femoral head should be repositioned immediately, as a true emergency. Supporting the thigh on pillows may partially relieve pressure on the femoral vessels [212] before reduction is accomplished.

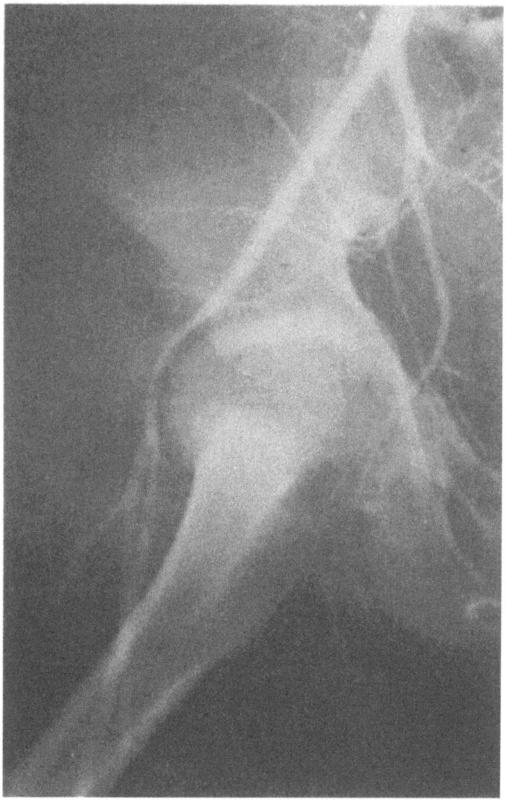

Fig. 4.13. Arteriography showing compression of common femoral artery by the head of the femur in a pubic dislocation – same case as shown in Fig. 3.8. (From Nerubay [339])

When the signs of peripheral arterial insufficiency do not rapidly improve after reduction of the dislocation, an arteriography (Fig. 4.13) or a digital arteriography must be urgently performed to provide an accurate diagnosis of the vascular condition [28, 90, 284, 382, 447]. When the pulse returns but the leg remains swollen, a femoral vein injury may be present [107] and should be diagnosed by venography.

Compression of the vessels usually subsides after closed reduction of the dislocation, provided it is done early.

Whenever the circulation has not improved after hip joint reduction, early exploration of the vessels, with the extremely useful guide of arteriography, is an absolute necessity. This is a surgical emergency and the vascular surgeon should proceed to perform treatment immediately according to the pertinent lesion. This early surgical treatment is the only chance to pursue a good prognosis in these instances; if this management is not accomplished, the future of the limb and the general condition of the patient are at high risk.

4.3.6 Open Dislocations

After careful debridement and cleansing of the wound, reduction should be achieved by the usual maneuvers.

Speed stated that no special effort should be made to suture the hip joint capsule [467]. However, Rinke and Protze used a homologous dura graft to repair the capsule due to a severe soft tissue loss in the anterior capsule [415].

Whichever the therapeutic protocol, the outcome was poor in all followed cases, with severe complications, including avascular necrosis, infection, and ankylosis. In some of the cases hip fusion was later performed.

5 Complications, Prognosis, and Postreduction Therapeutic Protocol

5.1 Complications

5.1.1 Avascular Necrosis

In 1919 Elsmlie described under the heading "Pseudocoxalgia following traumatic dislocation of the hip in a boy aged four years" [142], what appears to be the first reported case of avascular necrosis (AN) of the proximal femoral extremity (PFE) following THDC. Since then, numerous similar observations - 170, as far as I could determine - have been presented (Table 5.1 s.p. 119), leading to the general agreement that every child who has suffered THD may undergo this most severe complication.

However, the literature contains many conflicting opinions on this entity, for instance, the question about which cases should be considered as AN. A few authors have stressed the incidence of growth disturbances of the PFE following THDC [185, 190, 230], but without especially linking these changes with AN. However, interference with the blood supply of the PFE in a child should result in necrosis, not only of the epiphyseal ossific nucleus, but also of the longitudinal growth plate [26, 27, 60, 135, 251, 395]. While reviewing 145 cases of AN following THDC (AN-THDC), I could find that the anatomoradiological patterns clearly showed involvement of both these structures [27]. This is why I think that all those observations with radiological signs of compromise of the epiphyseal nucleus or the growth plate, or both, in a wide variety of severity and extension, should be considered AN-THDC.

A further point of contention in this subject refers to the name it should be given. Dysvascular or ischemic necrosis would seem to be terms preferable to AN to refer to vascular injuries in this traumatic condition because of the nature of the interference with the blood supply [350]. Other previously used terms have been osteochondrosis [94] and osteochondronecrosis [20]. Although AN is not the most suitable term on the basis of the pathogenesis and physiopathology of the process, it is interesting to note that is has been almost universally used up to now, and this is why I shall apply this term in this book.

5.1.1.1 Interval Before Diagnosis

AN-THDC has been diagnosed at various intervals following the dislocation, and consequently the opinion of authors differs concerning this interval. The interval between injury and development of roentgenographic AN has varied from 3 to 28 months [19, 27, 46, 63, 74, 85, 101, 236, 237, 351, 356, 383, 413, 420, 501], and in a statistical study on 145 cases [27] I found that the diagnosis was made in the initial 6 months after THD in ⅓ of the cases, within 1 year in nearly ⅔ of the cases, and in more than 92% of the cases within 2 years following the dislocation.

5.1.1.2 Symptoms and Signs

The symptom/sign complex is similar to that of Perthes disease and to AN following femoral neck fracture in children (FNFC). Following the injury and its initial treatment, there is usually an asymptomatic interval and the child becomes active and may even engage in sports. After a variable period which, as already stated, may range between 3 months and 2 years, some discomfort at the lower limb and stiffness at the hip reappears. As Kleinberg has described exactly [262], at the beginning these symptoms are present only when the child begins to walk. Soon the child finds that he cannot run or walk as well as he could previously. There is an increase in stiffness and pain, which may become constant. The absence of a symptom-free interval is exceedingly uncommon.

Physical examination reveals a limp of variable intensity, associated with hip pain, as well as an especially vicious attitude of the hip joint, with variable grade of flexion and adduction, while external rotation is not constant. All movements, but especially abduction and to a lesser extent internal rotation, are variably restricted and cause pain when passively promoted by manipulation. There is little or no local tenderness [262].

5.1.1.3 Roentgenographic Patterns - Physiopathological Basis

The radiological changes indicating AN-THDC follow different but constant patterns, which can be related to the sites and amount of involvement of the capital ossific nucleus and the growth plate at the time of the injury and reduction. These patterns appear to fall naturally into two distinct periods of childhood, i.e., younger children, usually less than 11 years old, and older children, 11 to 15 years old [27].

The irrigation of the growing proximal femur involves the zone of osteogenesis at the bony centrum of the epiphysis and the zone of chondrogenesis at the longitudinal growth plate [93, 106, 198, 349, 350, 395, 457, 492]. The diverse extents of involvement of each of these components are responsible for the wide variety of radiological patterns and clinical courses of AN-THDC.

Young Children. The initial *change in the capital epiphysis* is the radiographical appearance of increased density. The temporary arrest of enchondral ossification by ischemia leads to a relative diminution in size of the epiphyseal bony nucleus. However, the outer layer of the dome-shaped, peripherally growing cartilage, with its cells nourished by the joint fluid, continues to grow, but this cartilage is not ossified, which explains the radiological appearance of an enlarged joint space.

These changes are followed progressively by so-called absorption (Figs. 5.1, 5.2, 5.3, and 5.4). The necrotic bone is invaded by young granulating tissue, which further progresses to fibrous and fibrocartilaginous tissue. The resorption phase, with collapse of the invaded site with diminished biomechanical resistance, leads to flattening of the ossific nucleus. Although a definite fragmentation has not been documented in every instance, it has been described in a significant number of cases.

The following stage is that of reossification, with new bone being laid down progressively (Figs. 5.2, 5.3, and 5.4). Reossification continues until consolidation is complete, but ossification of the regenerating epiphyseal nucleus follows the distorted cartilaginous model [53, 265]. As will be shown, the ischemic lesions at the growth plate, leading to deformity of the metaphysis, will significantly contribute to deformity of the head in size and shape.

The varied roentgenographic appearance reflects the different grades of severity and the variable location of the ischemic disease, which ranges from very mild lesions with inapparent morphologic changes, to the most severe pattern with significant alteration of the size and shape of the femoral head. The last stage is remodeling, which will add improvement or deterioration to the shape of the femoral head, depending on the residual potential for growth.

The early signs of *damage to the longitudinal growth plate* (LGP) are usually subtle, and consist of radiological defects at the metaphysis. These are followed by either retardation of longitudinal growth of the femoral neck, or partial or total epiphysiodesis, i.e., closure of the LGP. Certain typical patterns of LGP damage could be found while reviewing the WS, viz., medial, lateral, or total damage to the LGP, the latter being symmetrical or predominant at its medial or lateral sides.

Variable grades of coxa vara result from the continued growth of the trochanteric growth plate (TGP) and the femoral neck isthmus (FNI), and from the relative or absolute retardation of the LGP. Whatever the pattern, a constant finding is widening of the femoral neck, due to continued normal growth of the TGP and the FNI (Figs. 3.17, 4.7, 5.4–5.6).

Medial damage to the LGP and continued lateral LGP growth lead to shortening on the medial side of the neck, with a consequent varus position of the head relative to the femoral neck and acetabulum. The head tilts deeply into the acetabulum [457].

Involvement of the lateral side of the LGP, with continued medial growth, leads to a valgus position of the head relative to the femoral neck and acetabulum [457]. There is progressive lateral subluxation of the head and head growth, which, together with widening of the femoral neck, leads to coxa magna [27, 457] (Figs. 4.7, 5.5, and 5.6).

Total damage to the LGP, when uniform, leads to symmetrical growth disturbance, with shortening of the neck as a whole, but without significant alteration of the head-neck relationship (Fig. 5.7). The TGP and FNI continue to grow normally, thus resulting in coxa vara. When damage to the physis is severe, shortening of the femoral neck is significant and the femoral head is flat, as seen in coxa plana (Fig. 4.11).

A correlation between the changes at the LGP and those of the femoral head in AN-THDC was found in a previous study [27]. If damage to the LGP and ossific nucleus has been mild, the PFE regains its normal shape and height. Whenever damage to the LGP leads to widening and shortening of the femoral neck, the development of the head is also abnormal, showing a clear parallelism with the LGP

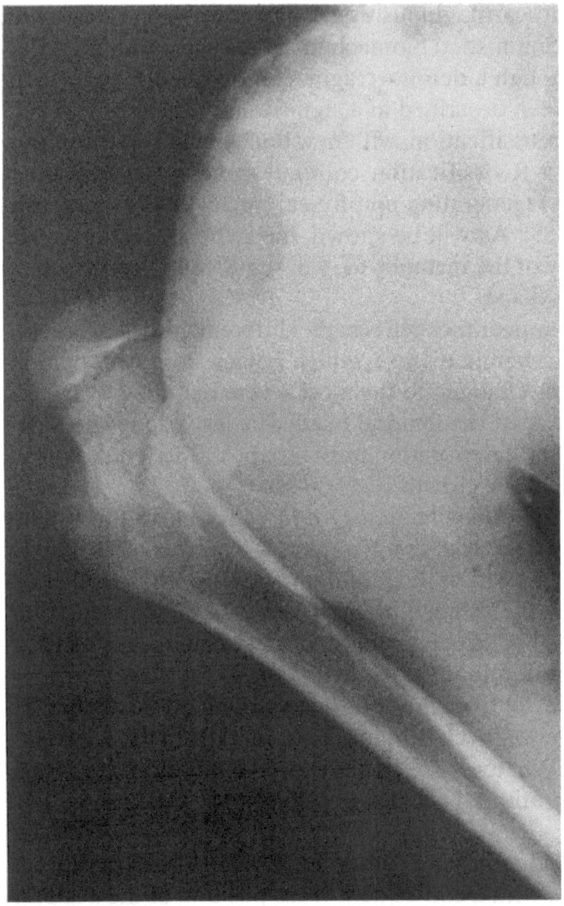
a
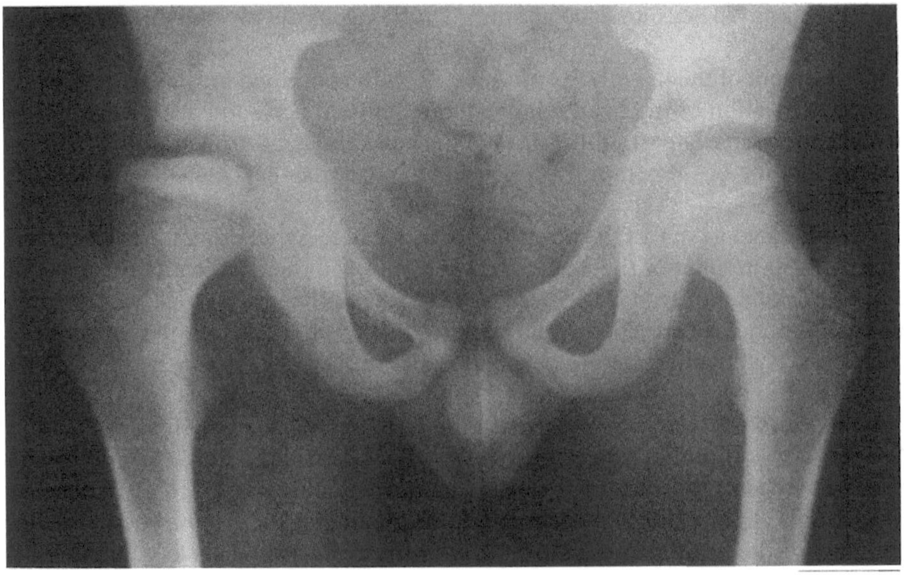
b

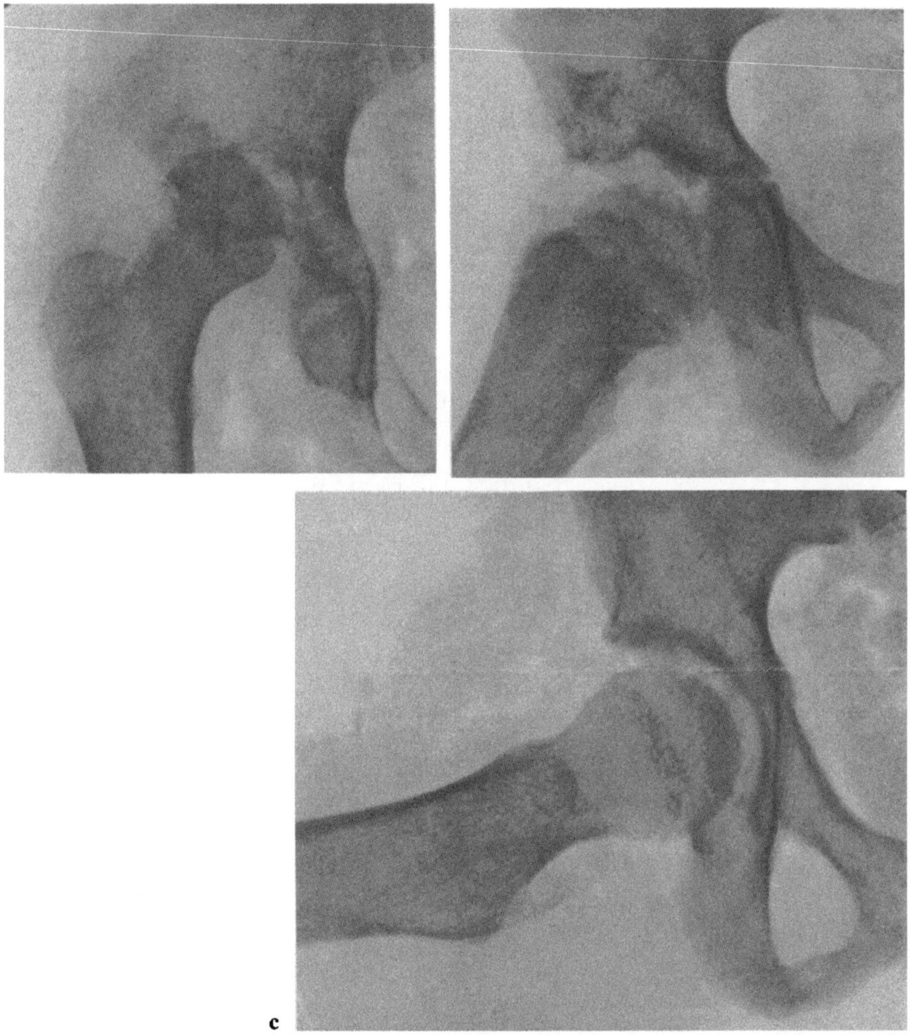

a b c

Fig. 5.2. **a** Anteroposterior view showing posterior dislocation of right hip in a 7-year-old girl, following an automobile accident. Dislocation reduced by open procedure 3 months later. **b** Six months later roentgenogram shows cystic changes within the head of the femur and irregularity of the articular surface of the head. **c** Condition 48 months later: almost complete reversal of changes and restoration of the normal architecture of the head. (From Freeman [168])

◁ **Fig. 5.1.** **a** True cross-table radiogram showing retroacetabular dislocation of right hip in an 8-year-old boy, following a fall off a tree. Closed reduction was performed 3 days later – diagnosis initially missed. **b** Five months later, there is condensation of the capital epiphysis, with collapse, and small areas of resortion

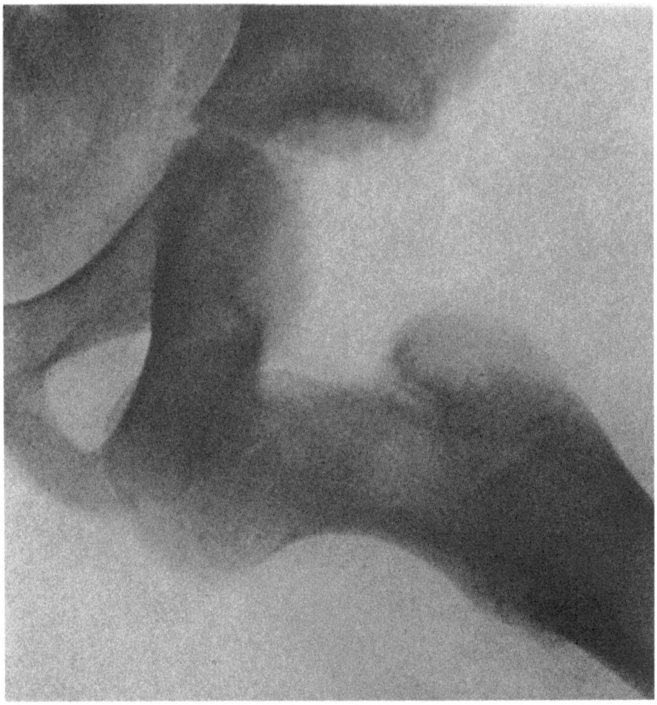

a

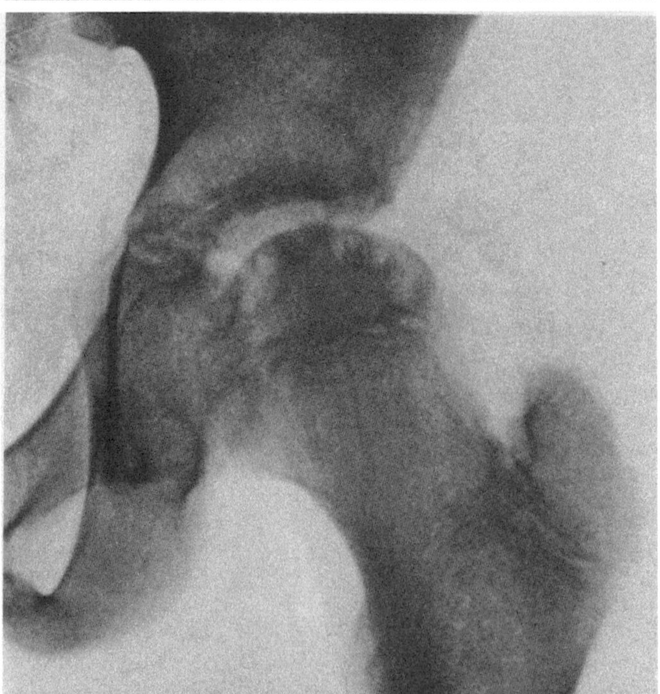

b

Fig. 5.3. **a** Obturator dislocation of left hip in a 12-year-old boy. **b** Roentgenogram after 15 months showed areas of replacement about the periphery of the head, while the remaining central head portion was extremely dense. **c** Anteroposterior view 22 months later showed complete restitution of the osseous center, except for several linear streaks of necrotic bone. **d** Roentgenogram after 6

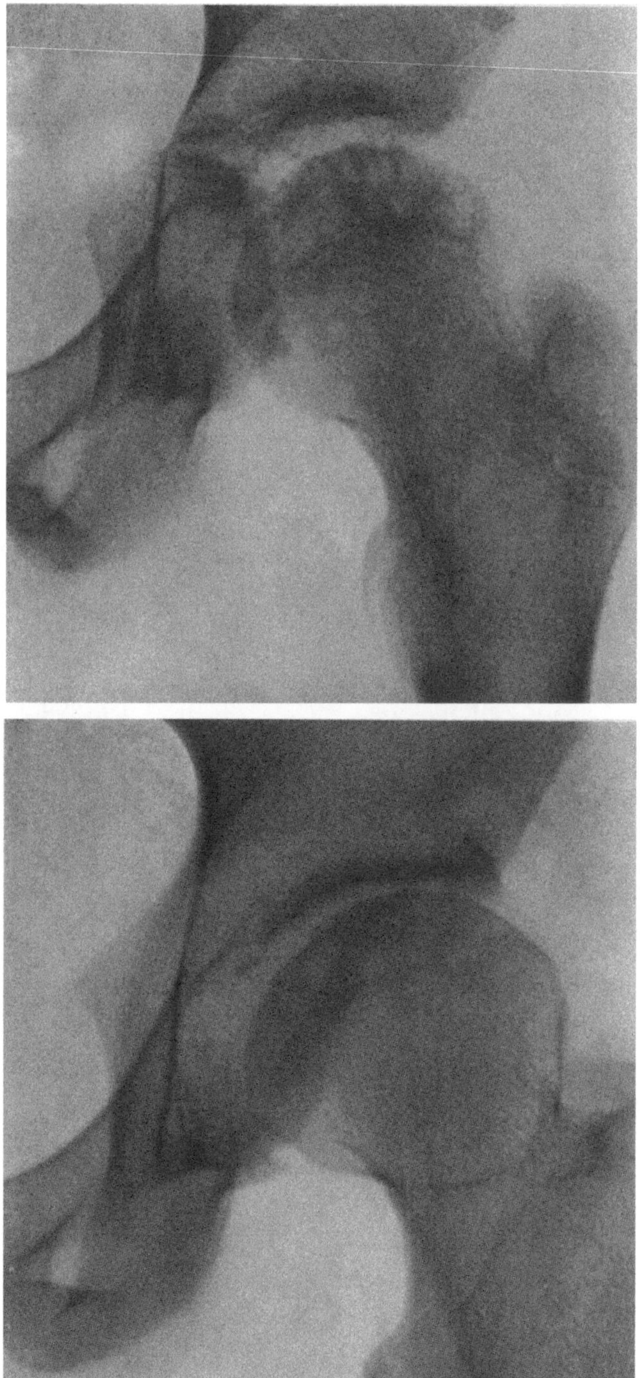

c

d

years and 2 months revealed a flattened but smooth head with maintenance of the joint space; no secondary arthritis. *Note:* Even though this was a 12-year-old male, the changes were most similar to those usually occurring in younger children. (From Banks [17])

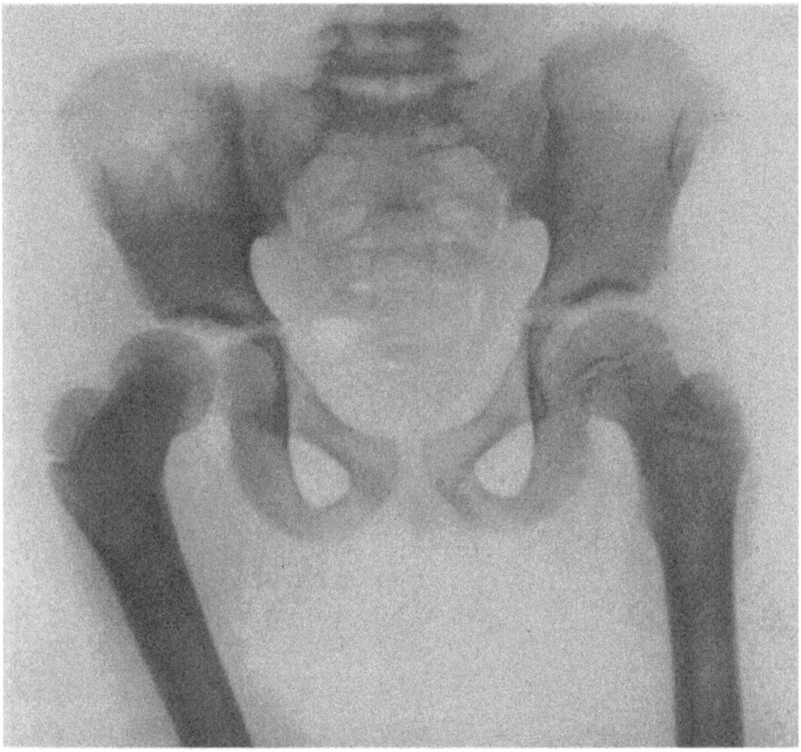
a
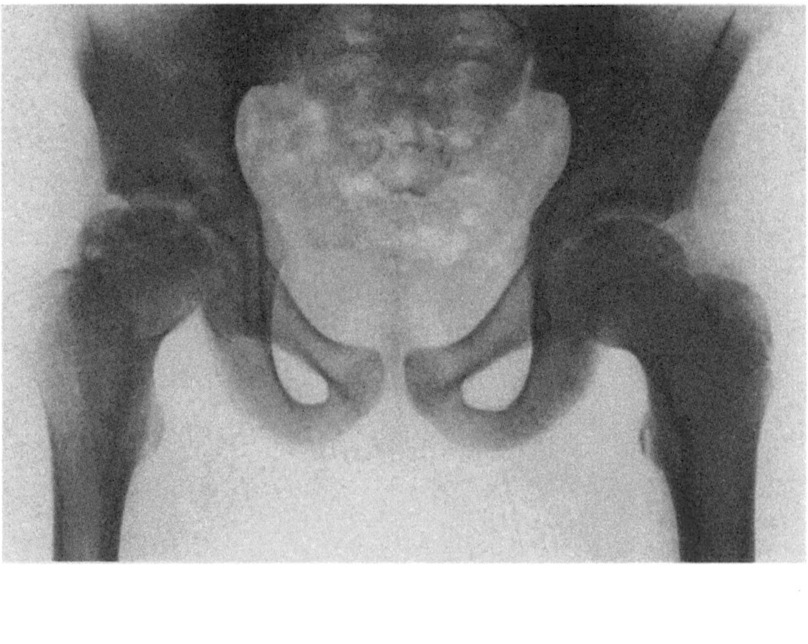
b

c

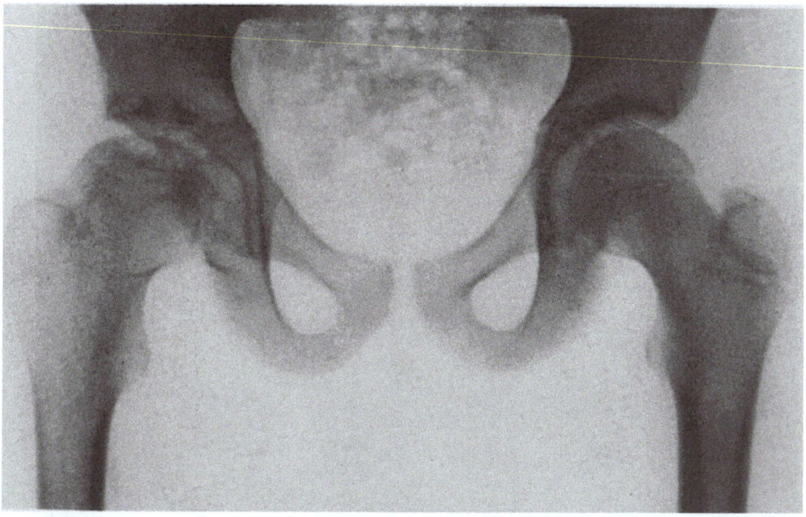

Fig. 5.4. a Roentgenogram showing posterior dislocation of the right hip in a 10-year-old boy after an automobile accident. Reduction after 8 days. Thirteen months later: limp and discomfort in the right hip and thigh. **b** Twenty-eight months after the injury: typical flattening of the femoral head with irregular areas of condensation and rarefaction. **c** Thirty-four months after the injury: the surface of the epiphysis is approaching a more normal curve and the density returning to normal. Note the broadened femoral neck and overgrowth of the head. Clinically, the patient had a complete range of painless motion and was symptom-free. (From Goldenberg [189])

changes. Thus, the deformities of the femoral head in children undergoing AN correlate with the physeal damage [27, 135, 198, 251, 457]: "this role of the physis is critical in establishing patterns of involvement" [60]. These changes (varus or valgus tilt of the head, coxa magna, coxa plana, etc.) are dynamic, they progress and even modify during the skeletal growing period.

Concerning acetabular changes, the acetabular development follows the alternative deformity of the PFE, probably as a result of their adaptative interrelationship [27]. An abnormal vascular femoral head does not supply adequate mechanical stimulus [251]. The triradiate cartilage allows an increase in the size of the acetabulum, while maintaining congruency between acetabulum and femored head [350]. Thus, deformity of the femoral head following AN will affect this acetabular/femoral head developmental congruence [350].

Radiological results demonstrate that growth disturbances influence the pathogenesis of sequela: nearly 95% of the reviewed cases in the WS showed coxa magna or coxa plana - to varying degrees - confirming previous findings [27]. Restitutio integrum, though extremely infrequent (2.6%), was also found.

The overgrowth of the femoral neck and head, known as coxa magna, has been considered a response of the PFE to a compensatory increase in its blood supply following the vascular insult [156, 167, 350, 406]. However, growth disturbances of the PFE suffering AN appear to play a more significant role in the development of coxa magna, especially in lateral involvement of LGP [27, 167, 457].

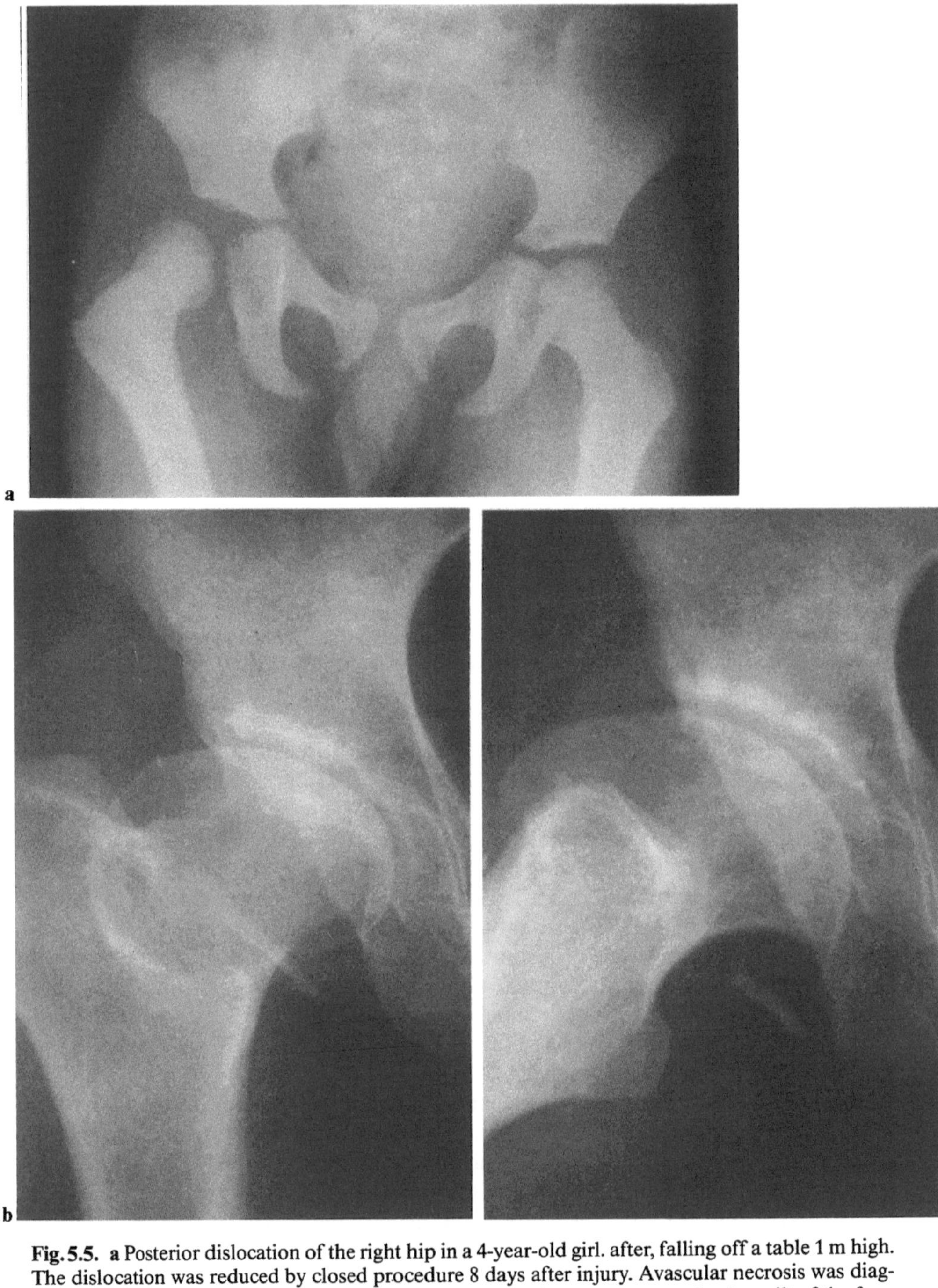

Fig. 5.5. **a** Posterior dislocation of the right hip in a 4-year-old girl. after, falling off a table 1 m high. The dislocation was reduced by closed procedure 8 days after injury. Avascular necrosis was diagnosed 20 months later. **b, c** Condition 31 years later: there is coxa magna and valgus tilt of the femoral head with respect to the femoral neck and acetabulum, as well as a wide and extremely short femoral neck. (**b** reprinted from Barquet [21])

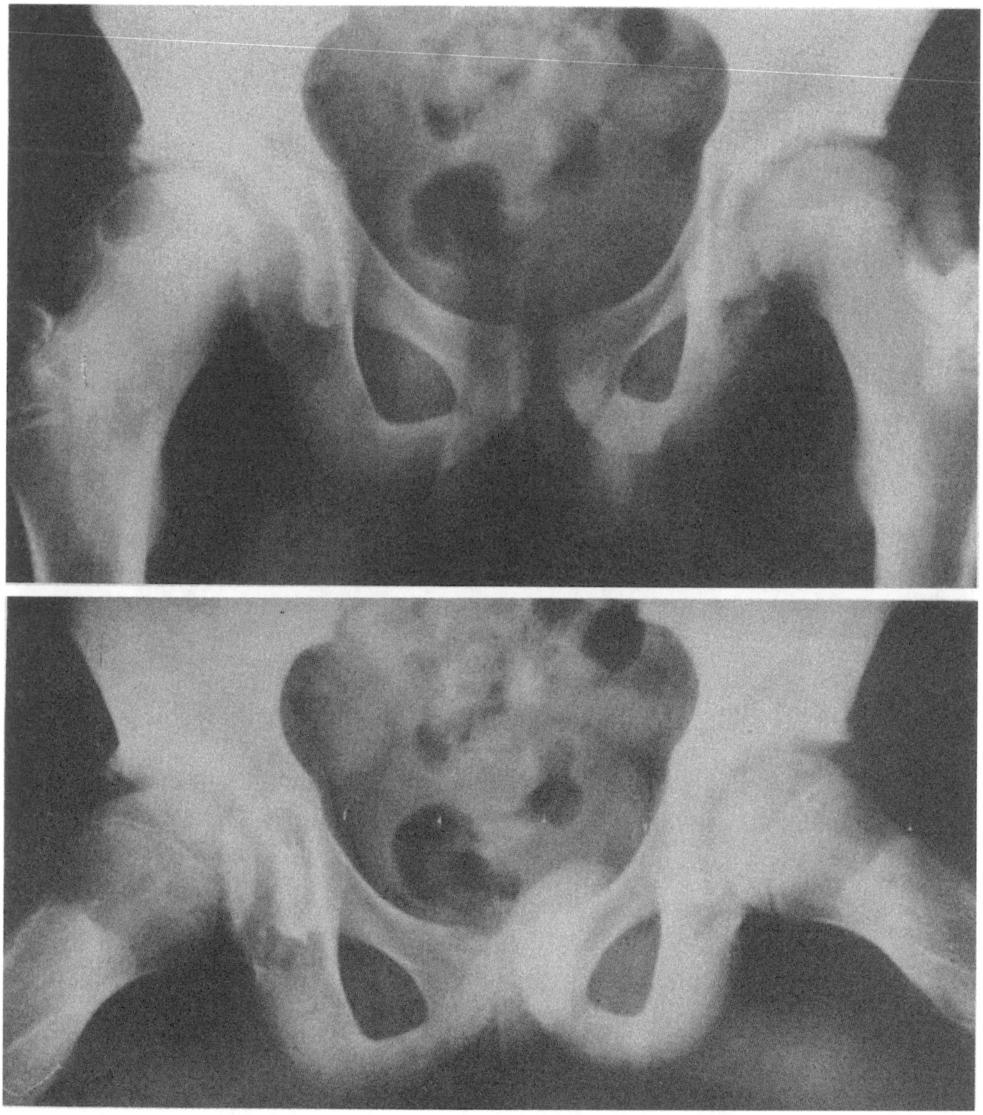

a

b

Fig. 5.6 a, b. Overgrowth of right femoral head and neck 21 months after traumatic posterior dislocation of the hip. (From Glass and Powell [185])

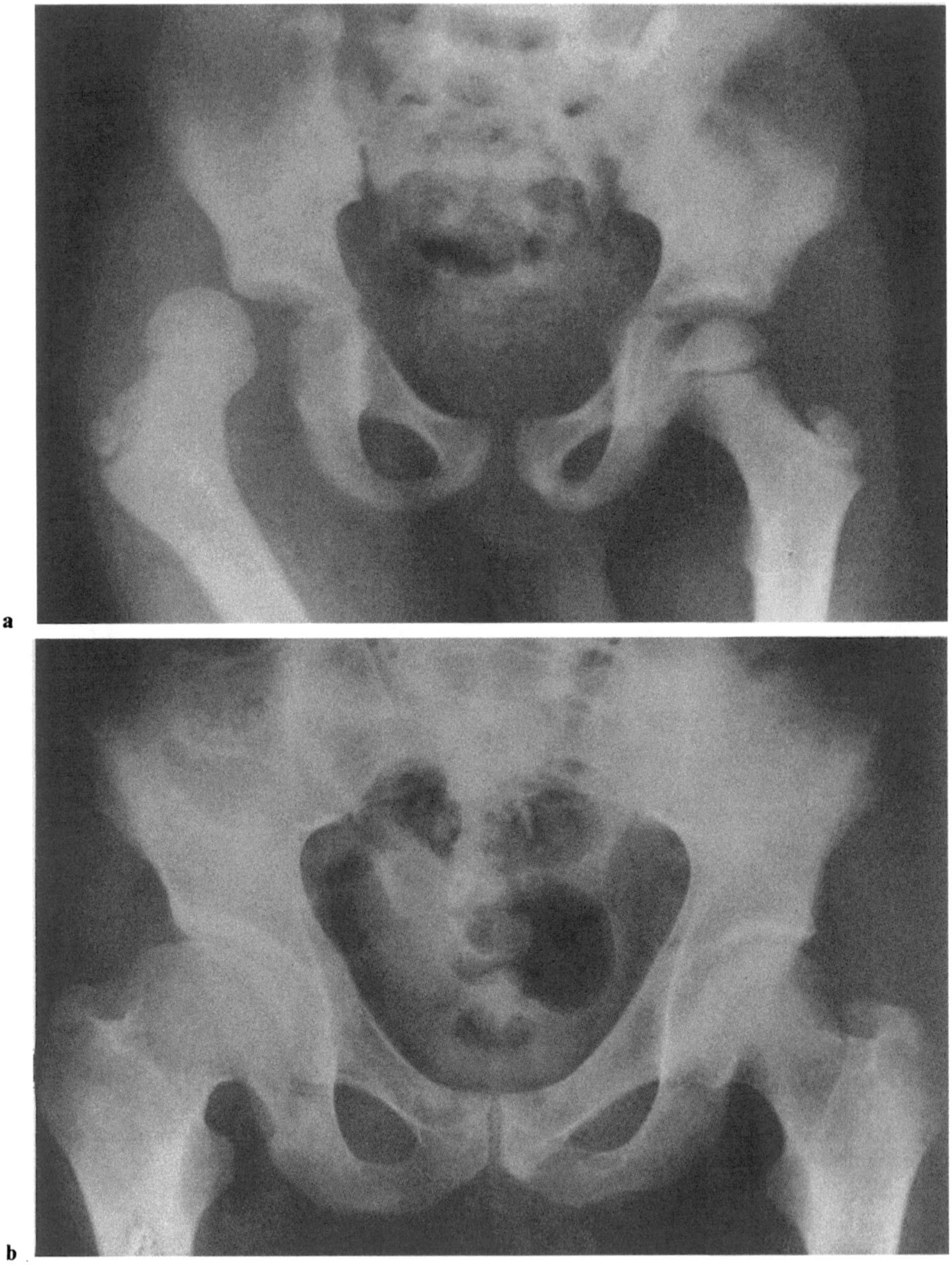

Fig. 5.7. **a** Posterior dislocation of right hip in a 9-year-old boy, sustained while playing football. Closed reduction was achieved 72 h after the injury. **b** Fifteen years later there is shortening and widening of the femoral neck, with enlargement and diminution in height of the head. No alteration of the neck-head angle. These changes would mainly result from symmetrical damage to the longitudinal growth plate. There is regular flattening of the femoral head. (**b** from Barquet [27])

The incidende of coxa magna ist extremely high (50%), with obvious different grades of enlargement (Figs. 4.7, 5.5, and 5.6). Coxa plana, with significant diminution of the height of the head, and significant shortening and widening of the femoral neck, occurred with an incidence of more than 40% [27] (Figs. 4.11 and 5.7).

Older Children. The incidence of growth disturbances in this age group is usually mild or even absent. Changes are mostly restricted to the femoral head, i. e., a similar pattern to that occurring in AN of the femoral head in adults [27, 284] (Figs. 3.9, 3.18, and 5.8). The radiological changes follow, as in adults, several phases [146, 158]: (a) nondeformed femoral head, but with areas of increased density and cysts; (b) depression of the subchondral cortex of the head, and greater areas of increased and decreased density throughout the head; (c) magnification of the signs found in (b), and defect in the head with collapse and irregularity; and (d) magnification of the signs found in (c), narrowing of the joint space, and signs of post-traumatic arthritis of the joint.

While reviewing the WS, I found precocious narrowing or obliteration of the joint space to occur with a significant incidence - higher than 50% - i. e., a rapid progression to phase (d) in nearly half of the cases of AN-THD in older children.

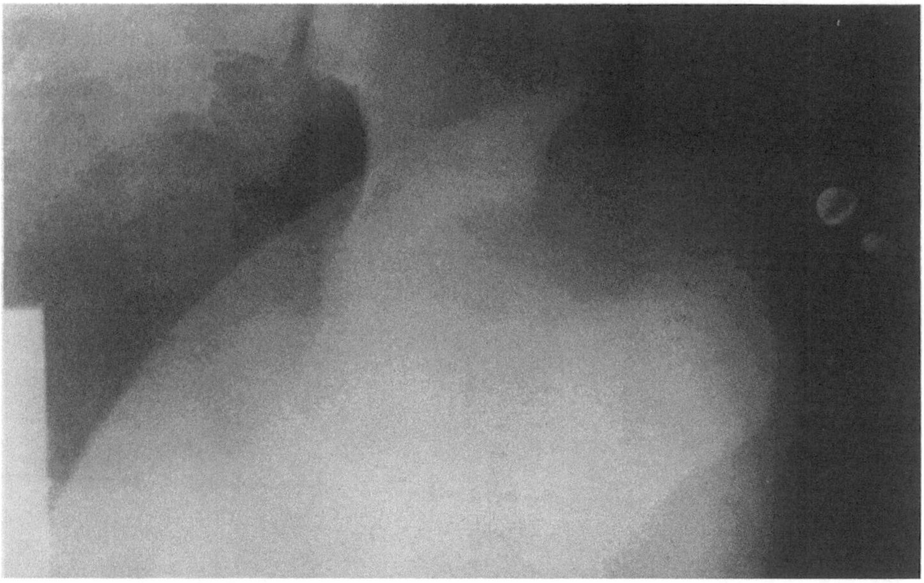

Fig. 5.8. **a** Posterior ischiatic dislocation of left hip in a 14-year-old girl, after an automobile accident. Closed reduction was achieved 2 days later. **b–e** see pp. 90–91

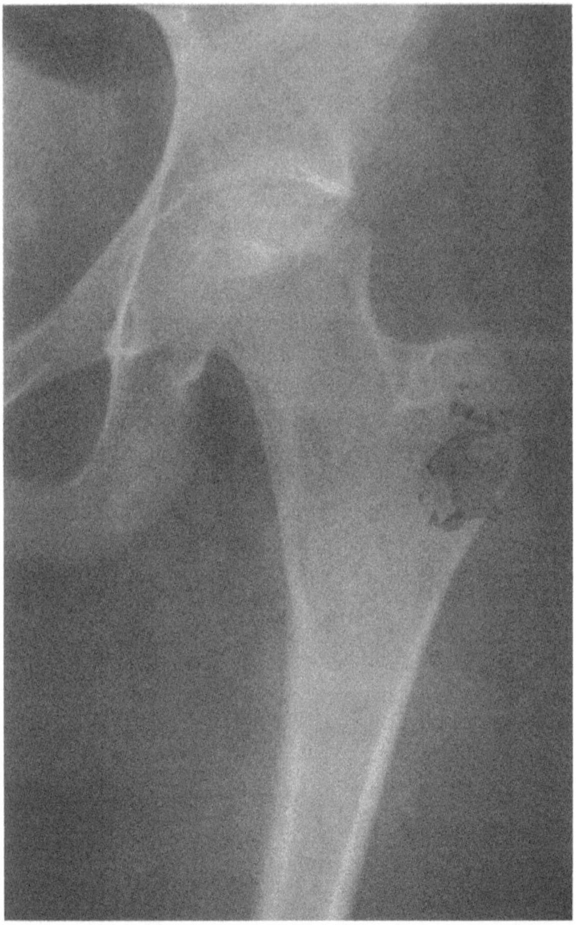

b

Fig. 5.8. b, c Twenty months after the injury there is evidence of avascular necrosis of proximal femoral extremity, with changes restricted for the most part to the femoral head, resembling those occurring in adults.

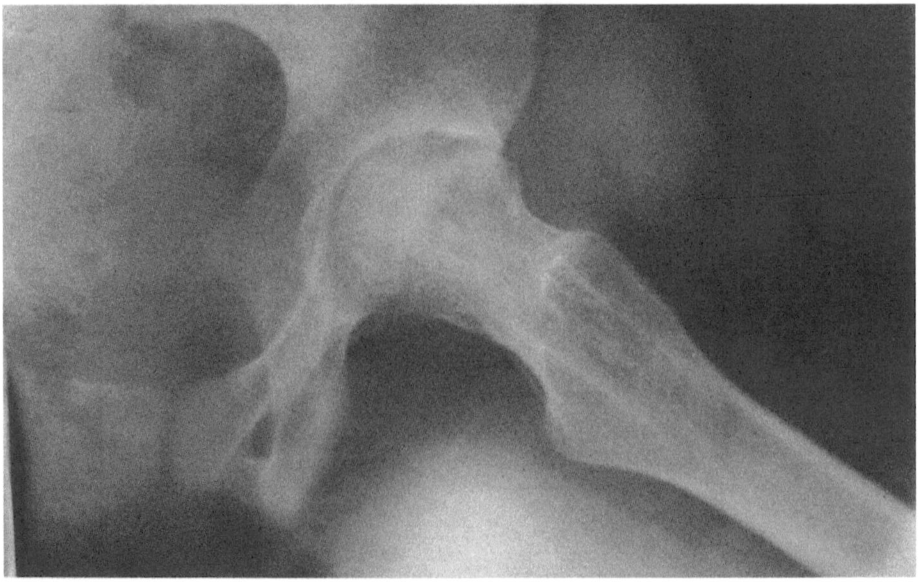

c

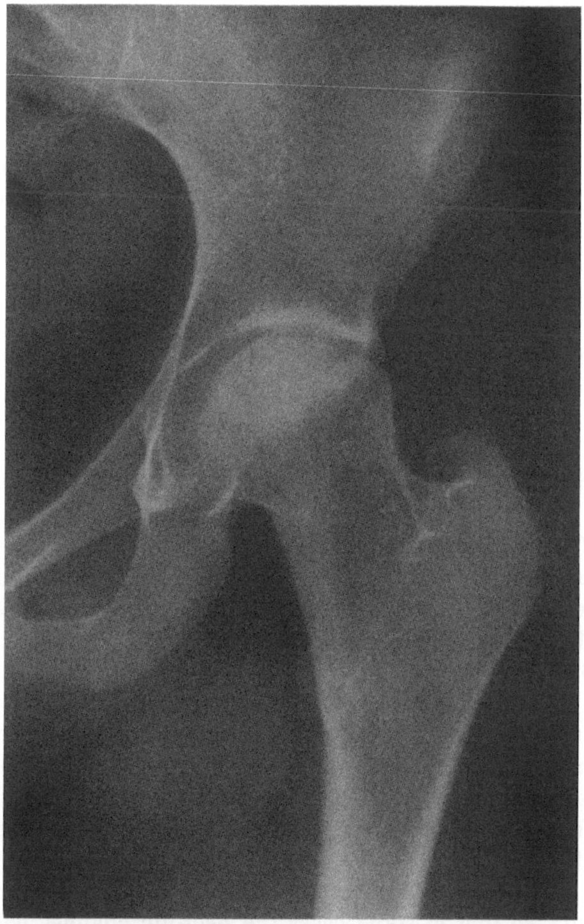

d

Fig. 5.8. **d, e** Condition 5 years after the injury. There is further alteration of the femoral head; narrowing of the joint space, although still not significant, is already present

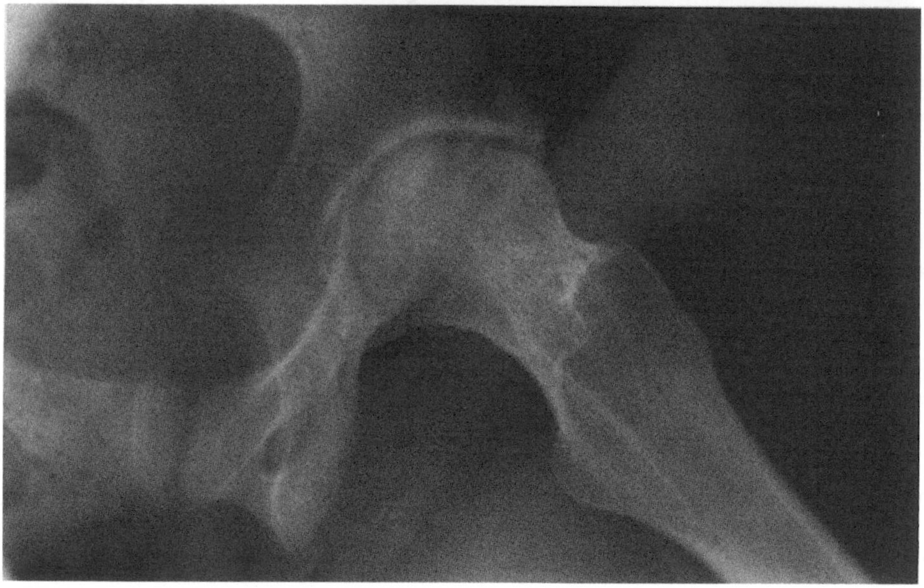

e

5.1.1.4 *Bone Scintiscan*

The interval within which AN-THDC appears on the clinical and radiological scene may extend up to 2 years, as previously shown. However, the advent of radioisotopes as a diagnostic tool has provided the possibility of early detection of a decrease in the vascularity of the PFE. A bone scan with technetium 99-m sulfur colloid or a bone marrow scan performed shortly after the dislocation should determine - with a 95% certitude index - those cases with initial ischemia, and would be of diagnostic and prognostic significance [27, 118, 236, 319] (Fig. 5.9).

A child who has suffered a dislocated hip should not only have an early scan, but also subsequent scans at 3, 6, and 12 months after the injury for careful evaluation of the vascular status of the hip [236, 350].

5.1.1.5 *AN-THDC and Other AN of the PFE in Children*

There are controversies about similitudes between AN-THDC and Perthes disease or other post-traumatic AN of PFE in children. There is a significant trend of opinion which considers the radiological patterns of AN-THDC to be very similar to those seen in Perthes disease [17, 19, 43, 48, 74, 101, 113, 142, 189, 262, 281, 341, 373, 382, 396, 410, 448, 517].

On the other hand, Haliburton et al. have stated that "Perthes disease differs fundamentally from AN-THDC: in the latter condition the epiphyseal plate may be normal and replacement of the epiphysis can occur in a surprisingly short time with adequate treatment" [208]. Chung has considered both entities to differ because the fragmentation and regeneration stages of Perthes disease do not occur after THDC [107].

However, in Perthes disease there is also great variation in the severity of ischemia, so that in some cases the necrotic changes will have completely cleared in 6-9 months [198, 466]. In addition, while reviewing the WS, I found further documentation confirming that there were numerous cases showing a stage of fragmentation in AN-THDC [17, 27, 43, 168, 172, 189, 341, 396, 410], and besides, it should be considered that not all observations have been documented or presented in their entirety.

While evaluating 145 cases of AN-THDC [27], I had found that "in younger children the radiologic changes of AN-THDC are similar to those of Calvé-Perthes disease in most of its features ... in older children between 12 and 15 years of age, the radiologic changes resemble AN of the femoral head in adults, as the potential of the growth plate has diminished a great deal." Similar opinions have been recorded from the literature [17, 284, 351, 476]. Ogden has considered comparisons of AN-THDC to Perthes to be inappropriate, because one is a more chronic type of condition, although the roentgenographic patterns are often similar in comparable age groups [351].

Elsmlie had found that the changes in his case were similar to those in children with AN following "reduction" of congenital dislocation of the hip [142]. I have found comparable facts, and these do not differ basically from those of Bucholz and Ogden [60] and Kalamchi and MacEwen [251].

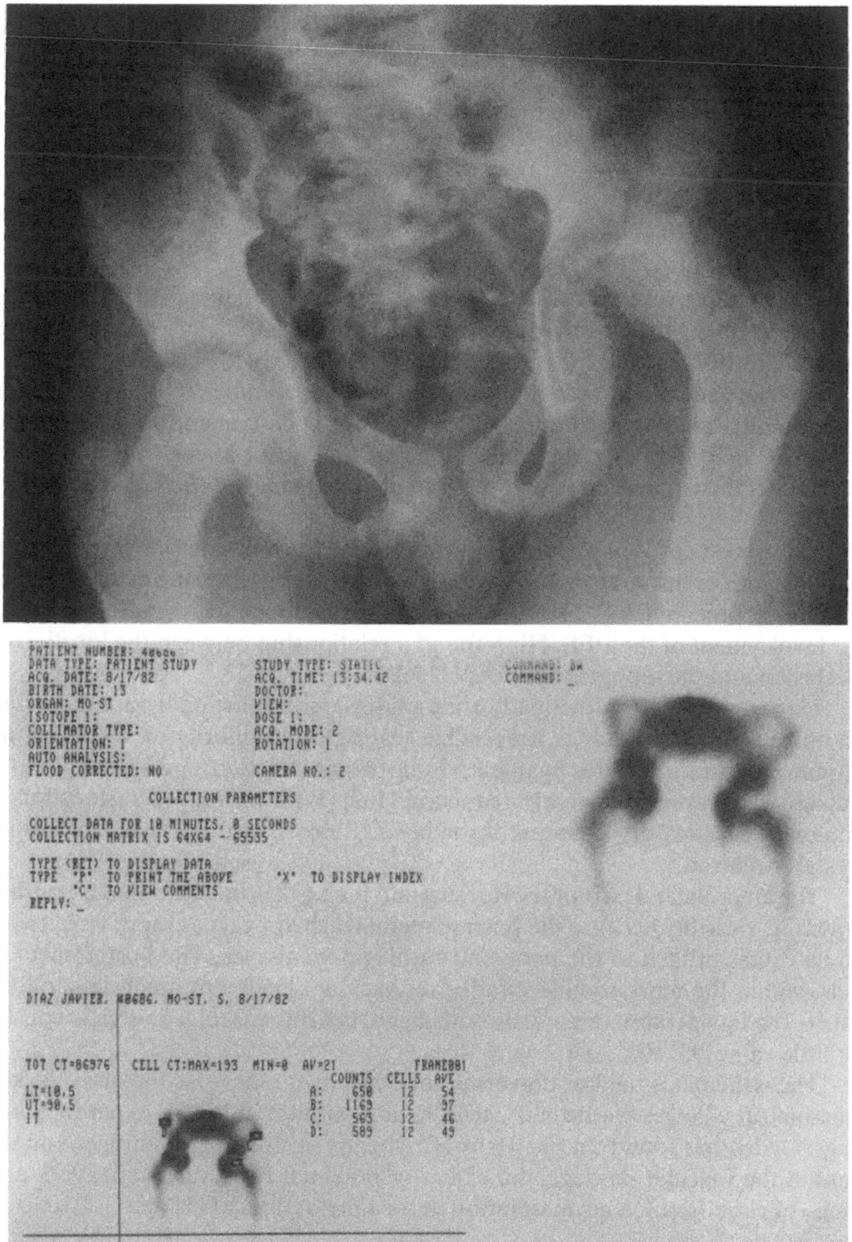

a

b

Fig. 5.9. **a** Posterior dislocation of left hip in a 12-year-old boy, after a traffic accident. Closed reduction was achieved 30 h later. **b** Four days after the injury the bone marrow scintiscan shows diminished density of isotope at the left proximal femoral end, indicating less vascularity than on the right side. (Courtesy of P. de Pena)

There is diversity of opinion concerning the relationship between AN-THDC and AN following femoral neck fractures in children. Certain authors have found certain similitudes [316, 337, 343, 476], and others such as Boitzy [53] and Ratliff [408], point out that several patterns of both these conditions are very different from one case to another.

5.1.1.6 Etiopathogenesis

The essential mechanism responsible for AN-THDC is damage to the extraosseous vessels supplying the epiphyseal and physeal region at the time of injury and reduction [27, 94, 103, 113, 132, 201, 226, 237, 242, 351, 385, 412, 434, 438, 455, 501]. The approximate site of vascular injury would be at the entrance of the vessels from the anastomotic ring into the bone, and so bypasses collateral anastomotic compensation [132, 282]. However, the series of events that occur after dislocation and how they affect the circulation within the proximal extremity of the femur are unknown [132].

The genesis of AN should be attributed to torsion, compression, elongation, tearing, and/or thrombosis of the vessels, which occur when the head is dislocated. The development of AN-THDC depends on the amount and duration of the vascular involvement of the PFE. Hipp found a relationship between the location of the occlusion and the topography of AN [266].

Duncan and Shim described, using rabbits, with functional vascular similarity to humans, injuries such as irreversible tearing of a minority of vessels along the ruptured capsule and teres ligament. Compression, traction, and spasm of the intact vessels were reversed by early reduction [132]. With prolonged dislocation, post-traumatic inflamatory changes, thrombosis, fibrosis, and occlusion of additional vessels occurred.

The anterolateral part of the nucleus and the LGP is most commonly or severely involved, possibly because the posterolateral leach appears as more vulnerable due to its course affixed to the bone and cartilaginous tissues. The posteromedial vessels, within the more mobile inferior retinaculum [350], are much less vulnerable [466]. The ligamentum teres is also damaged, but this vascular source is considered of little value [93, 106, 305].

The ischemia is neither universal nor definitive; otherwise the above described anatomical changes would not occur, a view supported by the experimental findings. Ogden has found that patterns of ischemic necrosis are contingent on the extent of the vascular damage, the extent of potential for revascularization, and the stage of chondro-osseous maturation at the time of injury [351].

5.1.1.7 Other Factors

There are controversies about factors influencing the development of AN-THDC. Previous analyses of available data in series of cases where AN developed, in order to find common denominators, are scanty [208, 370]. I performed a statistical evaluation in 1982, analyzing 145 cases of AN-THDC together with 267 THDC followed for at least 2 years without undergoing AN [26], and although further cases have been collected, their inclusion did not modify my previous findings, which are as follows:

Age. Younger children (under 6 years of age) show the lowest risk of developing AN-THDC [26, 61, 103, 107, 172, 192, 211, 351, 370, 420, 471]. There is something like a protection against AN in this age group. The incidence of AN increases with the child's age at the time of injury [26, 107], reaching its maximum in children between 11 and 15 years of age [26, 103, 192, 471].

The anatomical type of blood supply to the PFE in the different age periods of childhood would explain this influence of age to a large extent. The frequent mild causative trauma of THD in younger children would be another reason. There is a further argument, as shown by Ogden [351]: the age-related differences in the incidence of AN would depend on the volume of the ossification within the capital femoral epiphyseal cartilage. The greater the mass of bone at the time of dislocation, the more the normal vascular demand, such that it is unlikely to withstand prolonged ischemia; this obviously increases with age.

Sex. There is general agreement that sex is of no influence.

Severity of Injury. This factor has been found to strongly influence the incidence of AN-THDC [26, 91, 94, 107, 132, 304, 348, 351, 370, 376, 382, 383, 406, 413].

Variety of Dislocation. The incidence of AN after anterior dislocations has been considered low as compared with posterior cases [54, 94, 281, 289, 315, 382, 413], with the argument that the posterior vessels would escape injury by the anteriorly dislocated head [54, 315]. However, previous analyses [26, 236, 304, 471] and the WS have shown a similar incidence of AN in anterior and posterior dislocations. This may be explained by realizing that when the head dislocates forwards, the epiphyseal and physeal vessels are elongated and torn as well, as the distance between the posterior capsule and the femoral head is considerably increased [28]. In addition, when dislocation occurs and the head is propelled forward through the capsule, a further mechanism of damage to the vessels may be provided by the border of the capsular rent.

Type of Dislocation. FD are associated with a significantly higher incidence of AN, as well as other complications [55, 163, 326, 370, 383, 413, 420, 471]. The incidence of AN in dislocations with acetabular fractures proved to be three times higher than in simple dislocations, and necrosis occurred in all dislocations with separation of the capital femoral epiphysis [26, 31].

These figures do not differ from those occurring in adults, dislocation with separation being analogous to dislocation with femoral neck fracture. Duncan and Shim estimated the incidence of AN following simple dislocations to be 10%, and of FD to reach 35%, though this incidence may reach 70% in the presence of severe bone destruction at the proximal femur [132].

Interval Before Reduction. Delayed reduction is a most important influencing factor [12, 26, 42, 91, 94, 101, 103, 107, 111, 113, 132, 137, 155, 165, 267, 304, 322, 324, 348,

351, 356, 370, 382, 383, 406, 413, 420, 434, 438, 468, 471, 483, 501]. While reviewing 500 cases of THDC, Sterling found the incidence of AN to be 5% when reduction was accomplished within 24 h, and to reach 20% after 24 h [471]. AN-THDC has been said to be inevitable after an interval before reduction (IBR) longer than 12 h [102, 400, 406, 473].

I had found that if reduction was performed within the first 4 h the incidence of AN was 6%, if reduction was accomplished between 5 and 24 h it increased to approximately 13%, and after 24 h to approximately 66% [26]. Muller and Ganz had also stated that when dislocation was reduced within 6 h AN was rare, but after 8 h the incidence increased to 30%–50% [332]. Nevertheless, early reduction does not mean absence of AN.

This strong influence of the IBR is consequence of the recovery of the femoral head circulation enhanced by prompt reduction within a few hours. Conversely, delayed reduction is not invariably associated with AN [26, 383], although this fact is implicit in the given numbers.

Reduction Procedure. Undoubtedly, repetitive and brutal reduction maneuvers favor the development of AN [137, 483]. Some authors consider open reduction to be a factor favoring the development of AN [111, 113, 322, 475]. However, surgical procedures apply only to irreducible cases due to soft tissue or bone interposition, and to cases complicated with severe acetabular or proximal femoral fractures. Pietrafesa and Hoffman found that in dislocations with acetabular fractures types 2, 3, and 4, and in those associated with femoral head fracture, AN was evident in 22% of the cases, although this figure was reduced to 8% in Epstein's series when primary open reduction was performed [383].

Robertson and Peterson stated that no conclusion could be drawn as to whether open reduction adversely affects the outome [420]; similar conclusions have also been drawn by myself [26].

Postreduction Immobilization and Interval Before Weight-Bearing. There is little agreement about the influence of these factors. Some authors support the opinion that a short term immobilization of the hip after reduction favors the development of AN [68, 111, 468]. Some others consider this factor to be of no influence [113, 199, 236, 382].

A prolonged abstention from weight-bearing has been advocated to prevent AN [46, 68, 103, 111, 113, 137, 161, 172, 322, 361]. However, other authors maintain that this interval is of no influence [146, 370, 382, 385, 413, 420, 517].

I have previously found that none of these factors seem to influence the incidence of AN-THDC [26].

Recurrent Dislocation. As will be shown below, I found that complications in recurrent dislocation do not seem to depend on recurrence itself, but possibly on each isolated event [23], in agreement with Gula [201].

Conclusions. The age of the patient, the severity of the injury, the type of dislocation, and the inverval before reduction appear to be factors favoring the development of AN-THDC. It is not possible to conclude whether open reduction adversely affects the development of this complication. Postreduction immobilization and the interval before weight-bearing do not appear to be influencing factors.

The fate of the PFE seems to be determined at the time of dislocation and reduction [26]. Therefore, reduction should be performed as an emergency procedure, to diminish the risk of AN, a risk which nevertheless cannot be completly eliminated [26].

5.1.1.8 Incidence

Although most estimates of the incidence of AN-THDC range between 3% and 15% [19, 55, 58, 61, 68, 98, 107, 111, 134, 146, 161, 169, 201, 208, 236, 237, 242, 253, 267, 293, 309, 324, 326, 348, 370, 383, 406, 413, 438, 471, 483, 494, 519], these data are not exempt from criticism. First of all, there have been no definite criteria of evaluation, i.e., not all cases undergoing AN have been considered as such, nor have they been included in statistics in previous literature. I have found radiographic illustrations and information in previous reports which are compatible with AN as defined in this book, and not included in those reports as AN. Besides, AN may be diagnosed up to 24 months following the dislocation - at least from a statistical point of view. Therefore, theoretically only those THDC with a radiological follow-up of 2 years or more should be considered for statistical evaluation. Undoubtedly, this is not possible in a significant number of cases, and thus the statistical validity of previous evaluations is far from being "sans tache."

Second, there are several factors influencing the incidence of AN-THDC, as just analyzed. It is obvious that the frequency of AN will vary according to these factors, and this has been already emphasized in the literature. I feel there are different categories of THDC, with respect to the influencing variables previously mentioned, and the incidence of AN is different in each of these categories. In general terms, it can be accepted that the frequency of AN-THDC ranges between 3% and 15% in most cases, i.e., most cases are simple dislocations reduced within 12 h by closed procedures. But it should be born in mind that the incidence will significantly rise in FD, in cases resulting from severe trauma and in cases with delayed reduction. Finally, I endorse the opinion of Petrini and Grassi: "the incidence of AN-THDC cannot be definitely stated, for statistics and end-results are still not available on large series of cases" [376].

Comparison of Incidence of AN-THDC and AN-THDA. Here again, the literature is full of controversies. Some authors consider the incidence of AN to be greater in children [19, 55, 111, 169, 192, 242, 281, 382, 402, 444, 488, 501]; some others found the incidence to be about the same in children and in adults [309, 517, 519], and finally there is the opinion that AN is of lower incidence in children [46, 63, 94, 132, 163, 370, 376, 383, 413].

I feel this comparison is difficult to perform because there are many variables playing influencial roles in children and in adults. We cannot compare the incidence of AN in simple THDC with that of AN in FD in adults, nor can we compare those dislocations closed reduced in less than 4 h in children with those surgically treated (including internal fixation of acetabular fractures) later than 24 h in adults; each category would have to consist of comparable data.

However, if it is considered that THDC are most frequently simple dislocations, resulting in many instances from mild and moderate injuries and usually reduced by closed procedures within the first few hours, and that at least 60% of THDA are FD resulting from severe trauma, requiring supplementary open procedures in many instances, then I feel that as a general guideline one might accept the idea that AN-THD is, on average, more frequent in adults than in children.

Using a similar rationale, a higher incidence of AN following *femoral neck fracture* in children than AN-THDC results [53, 234, 351, 408].

5.1.1.9 Outcome and Prognosis

The final prognosis should be reserved until the patient reaches skeletal maturity [29, 258, 351, 370]. There is general agreement on this statement, since unanticipated changes may occur during the adolescent growth spurt and some changes are not manifest until then. Therefore, periodic radiographic review should continue until skeletal maturity, i. e., 18 years of age.

While analyzing the radiological aspects of AN-THDC, it was noted that the frequency of morphological sequelae is extremely high in the WS. However, it should be added that the radiological changes do not correspond to the clinical symptoms and signs in all cases. This condition of deformity of the joint, with narrowing of the cartilaginous space, persists without significant impairment of hip joint function during long periods in some cases.

Leg length discrepancy may also be the result of AN, as a consequence of collapse in height of the femoral head, and of flexion adduction deformity. This discrepancy after premature closure of the LGP secondary to AN will depend on the age at which AN occurs. As only 15% of the femoral growth depends on the LGP of the proximal femur, this third factor will be important only in young children.

Whatever it is, it should be noted that as a result of the high frequency of morphological sequelae following AN-THDC, a significant incidence of degenerative joint disease in the future life of these children may be anticipated.

And last but not least, the fate of the PFE, as previously indicated, is determined at the time of dislocation and reduction, and treatment of the complicating avascular necrosis, as will be shown below, plays only a relatively minor role. Therefore, prevention of AN is essential; early reduction of the dislocation is the only way to diminish its incidence.

5.1.1.10 Treatment

The management of AN of the PFE is still under discussion, especially because there is no efficient procedure leading to uniformly satisfactory results. In *young children* the deformities of the PFE following AN significantly correlate with physeal damage [27, 350]. Because of the significant role of the physis in the development of deformities, there are no therapeutic measures which have been shown to definitely influence the natural history of AN in children [27, 60, 251].

The principles of treatment recommended in the literature are similar to those indicated for Perthes disease, namely containment of the femoral head in the acetabular socket [20, 85, 236, 351, 457, 476].

Relief from weight-bearing has been recommended as a way to attempt to prevent osseous collapse during the early stage and revascularization period. This might be obtained in a number of ways: prolonged recumbency, sitting in a wheelchair, or by calpers, slings, or other splints. However, there are several authors who maintain that the results of such treatment are hardly better than the results of doing nothing [149, 198, 466].

There is general agreement that centering of the head within the well-covered acetabulum may minimize sequelae. This may be obtained by external splintage, but this involves a long-term immobilization and also the possibility of damaging other joints [198, 466]. Therefore, it seems that only surgical procedures may improve the mechanics of the hip joint. This refers essentially to centering of the head within the acetabulum by means of a corrective osteotomy - intertrochanteric or innominate - or even both, according to the case. Intertrochanteric osteotomy has the advantage of permitting correction at the joint and of the limb attitude [53]. Reorientation of the deformed head with respect to the acetabulum, or displacement of a necrotic zone serve to achieve weight-bearing in more favorable sites of the head; the attitude may be corrected as well. Extra coverage of the femoral head with an innominate osteotomy will take weight off the hip and help in preventing further deformities and early arthrosis [489 a]. The techniques of these osteotomies are not to be described in this book, and can be found elsewhere. Whichever it may be, these procedures, though useful, are only relatively efficient.

Premature epiphysiodesis of the TGP would be useful to restrain enlargement of this plate, thus diminishing the grade of coxa vara [350, 457]. Therefore, periodic evaluation of the hip would help in planning the adequate treatment for these children, in order to begin achieving better results.

In *older children* the pathological condition is most similar to AN of the femoral head in adults, as previously shown. However, total hip replacement should not be performed at this age. Therefore, surgical treatment, when necessary, should consist of intertrochanteric osteotomy. Arthrodesis appears as a second line procedure when there is major function impairment, as recovery and adaptation are possible, especially in young persons.

5.1.2 Recurrent Dislocation

Recurrent THDC (RTHDC) in a previously normal hip joint is indeed rare [12, 23, 103, 137, 179, 201, 230, 406]. Rigault et al. had stated in 1968 that in case RTHDC had ever existed, they had never observed it [413].

Since Choyce's publication on THDC in 1924 [105], collecting 4 "apparent" cases of RTHDC [96, 145, 180, 468], 28 additional cases of this unusual entity have been reported as such in the literature. However, 16 of these 32 cases do not appear to fulfill all requirements to be considered as true RTHDC: inadequate or unstable reduction of old dislocations, with reluxation occurring either immediately or in the initial few days or weeks [96, 145, 180, 486]; doubt as to whether the initial dislocation was ever reduced [189]; acetabular dysplasia [49, 311]; complete traverse hemimelia of the same extremity [222]; predisposing general factors, i. e., hypothyroidism and mongolism [172, 185]; initial dislocation with associated acetabular fracture [420]; second dislocation associated with acetabular fracture [230]; and insufficient data [294, 484]. Therefore, there appear to be 16 reported true RTHDC [12, 23, 136, 137, 168, 172, 179, 201, 228, 229, 261, 314, 338, 348, 370, 458].

The incidence of this complication in children would thus range near those numbers suggested by Lutter [295 a], i. e., 0.3%-1.2%. While analyzing the incidence of RTHD separately in children and in adults, a higher incidence in children results [23, 287, 295 a], as a similar number of cases of this complication have been collected in both adults and children, and THD in adults is much more frequent.

5.1.2.1 Etiopathogenesis

Morton stated that it is difficult to understand how recurrence could occur in children without bone dysplasia of the acetabulum, when fracture is so uncommon [326]. Several pathogenic factors have been previously considered as favoring recurrence. Severe trauma causing the initial dislocation has been mentioned. However, most of the original dislocations in observations undergoing RTHDC occurred after slight or moderate trauma, which has been previously found by several authors [23, 107, 201, 338].

Some other authors have supported the opinion that an increased tendency toward RTHDC results from delayed reduction of the initial dislocation [105, 137, 217, 287] and brutal reduction maneuvers [137]. Brief and inadequate immobilization has also been considered an important factor causing this complication - assuming an incomplete healing of the capsular tear [108, 137, 168, 228, 287, 351, 478].

However, a previous careful analysis of collected observations demonstrated that these factors do not appear to play any contributory role in the genesis of recurrence [23]. This is also verified by the extremely low incidence of RTHDC regardless of the method of treatment [107, 217, 230, 366, 458].

In 1964 Griffin suggested that RTHDC should be more likely to occur in the very young child [192]. Further reviews of cases undergoing this complication have shown that in the majority of instances children suffering RTHD were under 8 years of age at the time of the initial injury [23, 179, 201, 351, 458]. Thus, age may be mentioned as the only contributory factor to RTHDC, as far as statistics have shown, especially because THDC does not predominate in younger children.

5.1.2.2 Pathoanatomical Considerations

All RTHDC were posterior. Dall et al. [108] and Guyer and Levinsohn [205] each described anterior RTHD in an adult, but this variety has not been reported in children.

Minimal information concerning the anatomical basis of recurrence exists. Since few cases of RTHDC were surgically treated, pathological correlation is scanty [261], especially because these patients did not have a pathological lesion that was consistent [23, 458].

Several cases were described as having a saccular evagination or pouch arising from the posterior aspect of the hip joint through a tear or defect in the capsule, and filling or widening the interval between the short rotator muscles [12, 229, 261]. Analogous anatomical lesions were found in those RTHD also presenting a mild acetabular dysplasia [49, 311]. A saccular evagination through a leak derived from a detachment of the capsule from the acetabular rim throughout the entire posterior portion was found by Gaul [179]. Nelson found an evagination through a rent in the capsule, which included the labrum - which was separated from the acetabulum - together with a slight attenuation of the posteroinferior labrum [338]. There are other cases described as showing a herniation of the joint caspule from the posterior aspect with a tear [136, 458].

RTHDC may also be the result of a post-traumatic relaxed or attenuated capsule, without a tear [23, 137, 192, 458], possibly related to excessive capsular and ligamentous laxity inherent to young children [23, 294, 351, 358], in whom RTHD is more frequent.

5.1.2.3 Clinical Aspects

The average number of recurrences of THDC has been 1.68, with a minimum of 1 and a maximum of 4. The interval between dislocations has varied between 2 and 60 months, with an average of 17.6 months.

The causal trauma for recurrence is usually mild, a feature similar to recurrent dislocation of the shoulder. Symptoms and signs in each recurrence are similar to those of the initial dislocation, except for slightly severe pain in recurrences. In the interval between dislocations, clinical symptoms and signs are very mild, if present. Sometimes a sensation of hip instability has been described [382].

5.1.2.4 Roentgenographic Signs

The radiogram shows the typical signs of hip dislocation (Fig. 5.10). It is interesting to discuss whether X-rays may be useful in the interval between dislocations. A simple radiogram cannot show any abnormality, as the anatomical basis of RTHDC is represented by soft tissue pathology. Hip arthrography after RTHDC has been previously reported. Though not successful in certain instances [12, 229], it proved to be of diagnostic value in several cases [261, 338, 348], indicating the underlying pathology responsible for recurrence. Contrast material is introduced by the anterior via, and views demonstrate a collection of dye extending posteriorly from the hip joint as well as a posterior defect in the capsule [261, 338] (Fig. 5.11). A posterior leak disappearing over a 3-month period was also found [348]. Therefore, hip arthrography appears to be a valuable adjunct in providing diagnosis for RTHDC [12, 23, 137, 201, 338, 351, 458], and should be routinely performed some 4–6 weeks after recurrence has been treated, thus providing guidelines for definitive treatment of RTHDC. As the exact site of the tear may not be clearly demonstrated, Klein et al. recommend combined CAT arthrography, which shows the communication between the posterior aspect of the hip joint and the collection of contrast material [261] (Fig. 5.11).

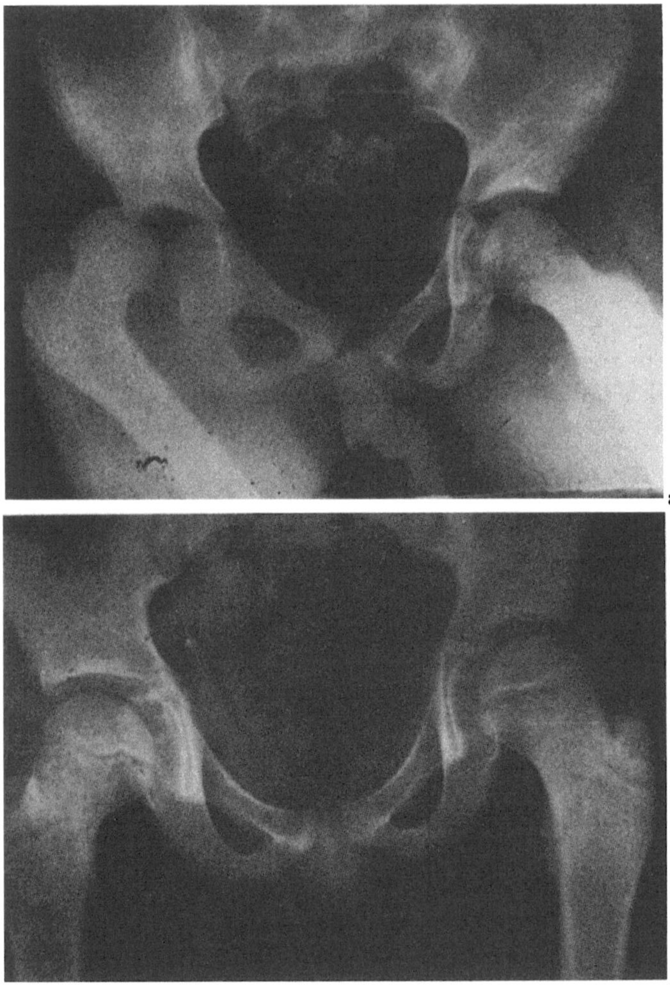

a

b

Fig. 5.10. **a** Posterior dislocation of right hip in a girl aged 7 years and 11 months, who fell from a wall ½ m high. There is no evidence of osseous abnormalities. **b** Condition after closed reduction 4 h later. **c** Recurrent dislocation of the right hip, 3 months later, while falling from a bicycle. Closed reduction performed 6 h later. **d** Normal hip 8 years later. (From Barquet [23])

5.1.2.5 Outcome and Prognosis

In previous reports the average interval between initial and final dislocation has been 2.5 years, indicating a logical minimal follow-up period of 2.5 years.

Among previous observations, only one child developed AN [168], and it was difficult to determine whether necrosis was the result of recurrence or of the initial dislocation. Previous analyses suggest that complications in RTHDC do not depend on recurrence itself, but possibly on each isolated event [23, 201].

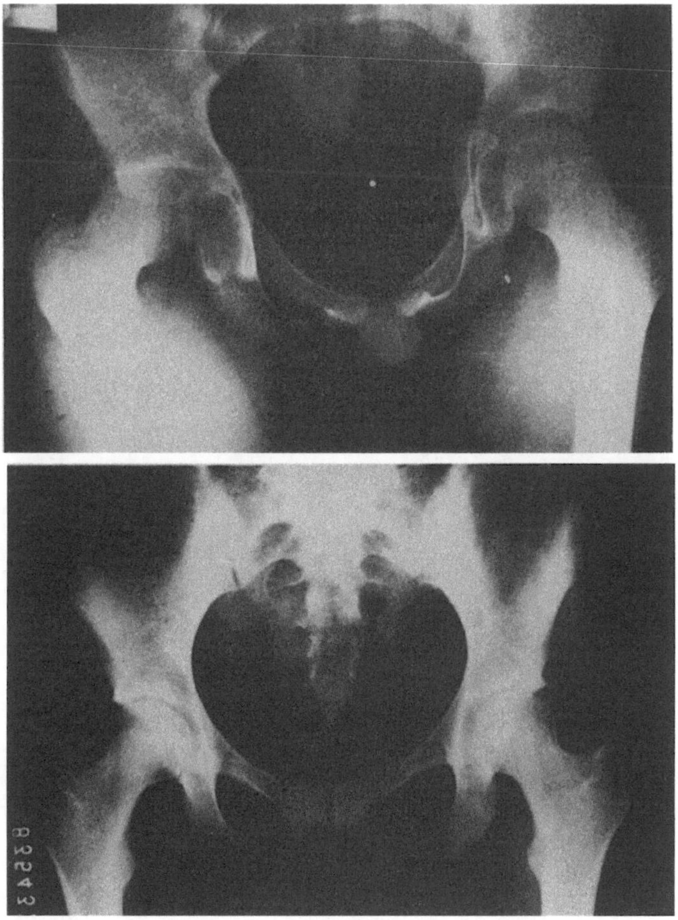

c

d

5.1.2.6 *Treatment*

Treatment of RTHDC has remained very much a matter of choice [229]. However, and in spite of the small number of reported cases, certain therapeutic trends can be suggested.

When arthrography shows a saccular evagination through a capsular defect of the joint, an excision of the pouch and a repair of the capsular defect should be performed [12, 23, 49, 107, 136, 179, 217, 229, 230, 261, 287, 311, 458]. The joint should be exposed in such a way that the entire posterior capsule may be easily inspected through a posterior approach [351, 458]. The acetabulum should also be carefully inspected. After excising the pouch, capsulorrhaphy should be done by overlapping and firmly suturing the defective lips in a "double breasted" manner [107], and with the thigh in neutral rotation or, better, in slight external rotation [49] to diminish the defect. An associated plication of the short rotator muscles has been recommended as a complementary procedure [49, 229, 311, 338].

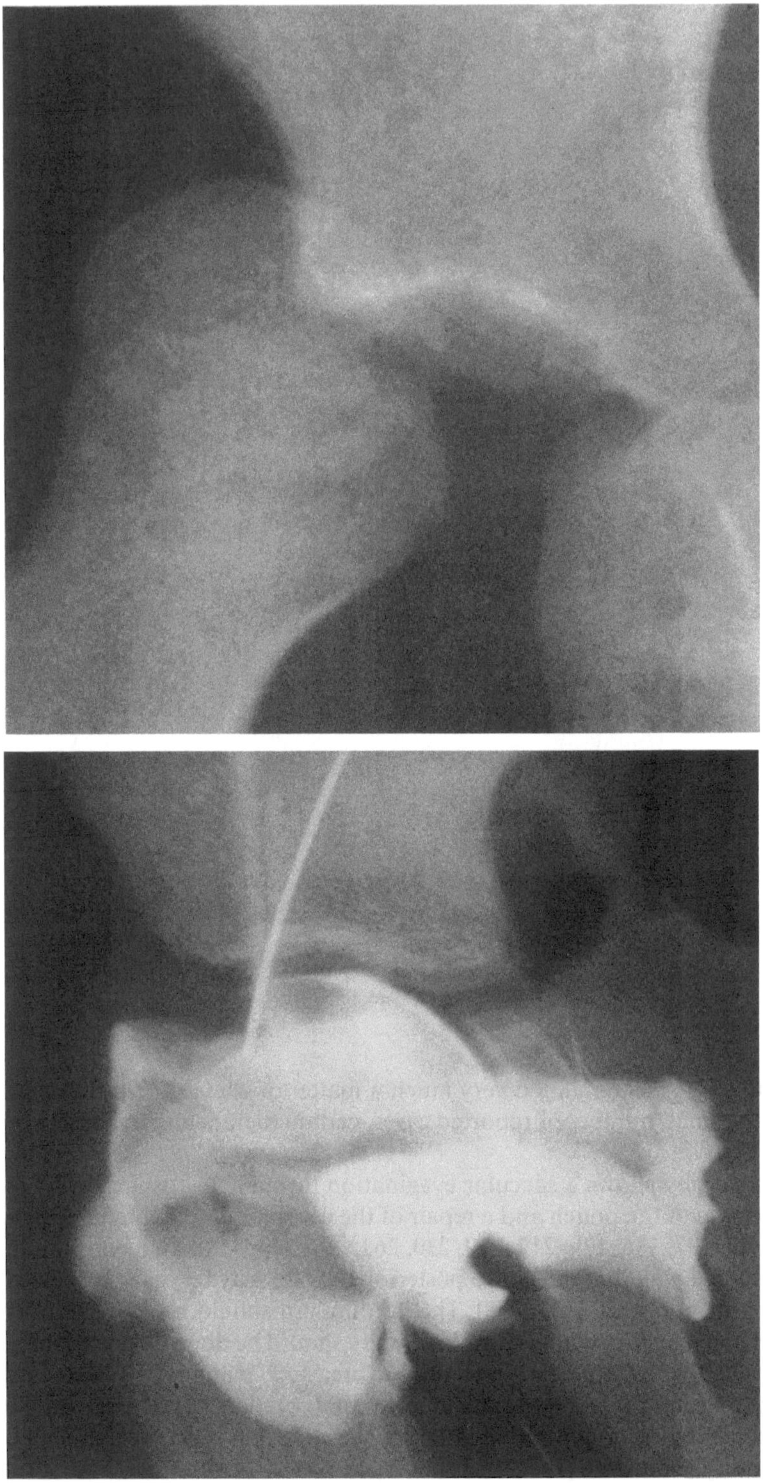

a

b

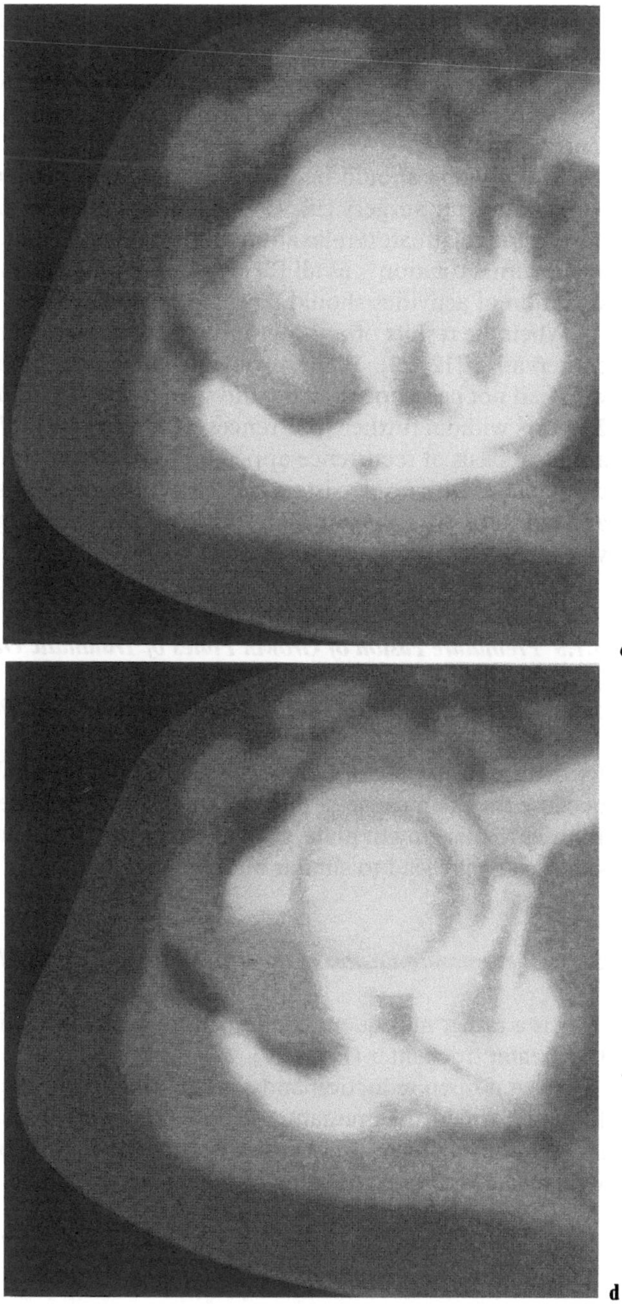

Fig. 5.11. **a** Admission film. Posterior dislocation of right femoral head in a 6-year-old boy after he fell off a bicycle. It was the fourth dislocation of right hip, all after minimal trauma, in 2 years. Closed reduction was accomplished. **b** Four weeks later hip arthrogram was performed: contrast extends posteriorly, but exact site of defect was not demonstrated. **c, d** Combined CAT and arthrogram localize site of posterior contrast leakage into muscles. No anterior component. The tear was subsequently confirmed and repaired at operation. (From Klein et al. [261])

When there is an associated detached or torn labrum, freshening and reattachment of the labrum to the osseous acetabular rim is recommended whenever possible [338]. Duyfjes used a concomitant iliac graft inserted into the posterior margin of the acetabulum [136], but no further reports with this procedure have been presented.

The hip joint should be immobilized with a plaster hip spica for a period of 6 weeks following surgery [12, 179, 311, 338, 458]. The limb should be maintained in the position of greatest relaxation of the damaged tissues, i. e., extension, abduction, and external rotation - as all RTHDC were posterior [107, 351, 458]. Progressive resumption of activities should be encouraged later on.

When the results of arthrography show no capsular defect, treatment should be conservative [12, 23]. While reviewing previously published cases, some patients who had not been operated on and who had been followed for periods longer than 2.5 years without further recurrences were found [23, 172, 314]. In such cases the anatomical basis of recurrence appeared to be a post-traumatic attenuated or relaxed capsule, but with no persistent defect. With growth this soft structure might tighten and aid stability of the joint [23, 294, 358]. Thus, no surgical treatment should be advised.

5.1.3 Premature Fusion of Growth Plates of Traumatic Origin

5.1.3.1 Premature Fusion of the Longitudinal Growth Plate

Premature fusion of the LGP has been thoroughly analyzed under the heading AN because the main cause of damage to this growth plate is precisely AN of the PFE. Injuries to this growth plate, such as partial or complete separation, compression lesions, etc., may lead to similar outcomes.

5.1.3.2 Premature Fusion of the Trochanteric Growth Plate

This is a rather infrequent complication, mainly resulting from fracture avulsion of the greater trochanter (Fig. 3.11).

Even if open reduction and internal fixation of the avulsed trochanter are carefully performed, the premature fusion of the growth plate may occur. Due to this fusion, and to the continued growth of the LGP, an elongation of the femoral neck with a valgus tilt, i. e., opening of the neck-shaft angle, will result (Fig. 5.12).

5.1.3.3 Premature Fusion of the Acetabular Triradiate Cartilage

Injuries to this growth cartilage, causing premature fusion of one or more of its arms, with further maldevelopment of the acetabulum [351], is a rare complication after THDC.

Dislocations of the hip with fracture of the acetabulum mostly occur in older children, when the potential for growth of the triradiate cartilage has diminished a

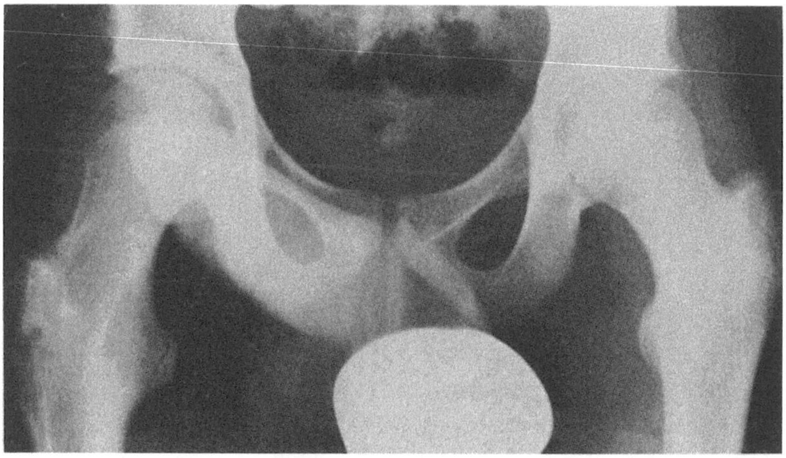

Fig. 5.12. Avulsion of entire greater trochanter accompanying anterior hip dislocation in a child 7 years of age led to premature arrest of the trochanteric growth plate and overgrowth of femoral neck, the latter due to continuing growth of the longitudinal growth plate, causing an elongated femoral neck and an extremely open femoral neck-shaft angle. (Form Ogden [350])

great deal or is absent. Thus, changes at the acetabulum in THDC mostly depend on fractures and not on premature fusion of this growing plate, as confirmed while evaluating the WS.

5.1.4 Heterotopic Ossification

There is no general agreement about the real nature of this complication, and consequently its designation has been different from one author to the other. Some authors call it myositis ossificans, as an analogous entity to that occurring in muscles in certain circumstances [351, 487]. However, it has been also found that ossification following THD occurs either at the muscles, capsule, and ligaments, or even at the interstitial tissues, thus receiving the name of heterotopic ossification [356, 420, 434]. Finally, there is the opinion of others, who state that it is not truly a heterotopic bone formation, but just a calcification without the exact bony architecture [498]. I prefer to call it heterotopic ossification (HO).

5.1.4.1 Incidence

When considering the incidence of HO in THDC it should be remembered that there are different degrees of severity of this complication. In a majority of instances the ossification is minute or mild. In addition, there are moderate bone formations, and finally only in the lesser percentage of cases is the extent of ossification significant.

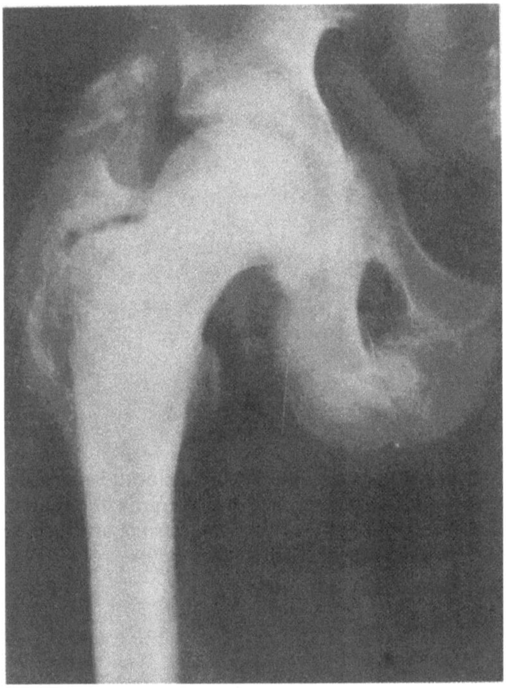

Fig. 5.13. Radiograph of right hip 6 months after anterior pubic dislocation with heterotopic ossification (same case as shown in Figs. 3.8 and 4.13); hip dislocation was associated with compression of the common femoral artery and laceration of the femoral vein; dislocation was irreducible due to a buttonhole tear of the anterior capsule and interposition of rectus femoris and iliopsoas tendons. Open reduction was performed early. (From Nerubay [339])

The presence of traces of mild HO at the soft tissues about the hip joint following THDC is not very infrequent. However, these are, in general, fortuitous findings while radiologically controlling the outcome of a hip dislocation. In certain instances, these HO are severe and determine functional impairment to a significant degree at the joint, leading in its more severe grades to a great limitation of movement or even complete loss of it (Figs. 4.10, 5.13). While reviewing the WS, I only found 19 cases of HO following THDC [39, 70, 185, 279, 298, 339, 365, 420, 441, 452, 465, 494, 512], but these include observations with the most minute ossification and without clinical influence. Among these 19 cases only 5 presented functional impairment related to HO which adversely affected the patient's outcome. The latter are the cases which in fact should be considered while analyzing HO, and their incidence is therefore extremely low (less than 1%) in the WS.

5.1.4.2 Etiopathogenesis

The pathogenesis of HO following THD has been related to hematoma and muscle trauma resulting from the injury [146]. Pidhorz and Mouterde implicate capsular avulsions as the pathogenic mechanism [382]. Pagano et al. state that HO originates directly from the traumatic lesions or from the prolonged muscular contracture [361]. Whatever the cause, there appears to be a neurovascular disturbance locally induced by trauma, with fibroconnective metaplasia, leading to the organization and ossification of the capsular and pericapsular hematoma [405]. I feel that for HO to occur there must be something like an individual predisposition.

Several factors are usually mentioned as favoring HO: concomitant head injuries [351, 517]; inadequate and repetitive - even brutal - reduction maneuvers, especially when performed without general anesthesia [101, 137, 487, 517]; delayed reduction [101, 137, 342, 382, 487]; dislocated hips that have been treated by surgery [146, 191, 382], especially when an acetabular fragment has been internally fixed; lack of immobilization [342]; passive, and forced postreduction rehabilitation maneuvers and massages [52, 101, 137, 199, 365, 382, 487, 517]; and early resumption of weight-bearing, when the hip is still painful [137]. In addition, it has been considered that HO are almost unknown in simple dislocations [517], and Epstein [146] and Gregory [191] have insisted that HO is most likely to occur when the injury is associated with a considerable hematoma.

However, careful analysis of the cases with HO from the WS has shown that none of these factors may be considered as significantly related to the etiology of HO, except for concomitant head injuries, which occurred in 26% of these collected observations.

It is possible that the potential influence of some factors does not show in this collected series because previous authors have emphasized the importance of avoiding repetitive and forceful maneuvers while reducing the dislocation, and because most orthopedic surgeons have contraindicated passive mobilization and massages while rehabilitating patients with injuries at their limbs, and this for several decades already. Brav [57] and Epstein [146] have also found that neither early active exercises nor early weight-bearing appear to be factors causing HO.

5.1.4.3 Symptoms and Signs

HO appears on the clinical and radiological scene as soon as 3-4 weeks following the injury [137, 434], and rapidly increases in a few months. Sometimes, the lesion and its indicating symptoms and signs undergo a mild regression, but without disappearing. However, in other instances, there is progression of HO, leading to the most severe types of the lesion.

There is functional impairment, which ranges from a simple antalgic contracture (periarticular muscles) to the significant limitation of the mobility of the joint [101, 356, 434]. This impairment is painful, and the pathological attitude of the limb may become fixed [356]. Weight-bearing in also painful. However, even marked ossifications can be present without subjective or objective symptoms [365].

Pagano et al. have suggested that if HO occurs at the muscles the clinical manifestations are relatively minimal and are not an obstacle to functional recovery unless they reach large dimensions. These authors have also stated that when ossification of the capsule and pericapsular tissues takes place, significant functional consequences are more frequent [361].

Gregory has indicated that a clue in determining which patients may develop HO is hemorrhage - marked swelling after dislocation means hemorrhage [391]. However, this fact was not definitively demonstrated.

5.1.4.4 Radiological Signs

Minute or mild HO - most cases - appear on the radiograms as traces of ossification either at the tip or above the greater trochanter, in the region of the lesser trochanter, or around the acetabular rim. The size of the ossification is small and, as previously stated, these HO are not associated with clinical symptoms or signs.

The larger forms, i.e., significant HO, appear laterally or medially with respect to the acetabular rim as a calcified structure which prolongs the rim [356, 434]. When they are lateral to the rim, they appear as an ossified bridge which joints the acetabular roof to the greater trochanter (Figs. 4.10 and 5.13). *When they are medial,* they look like a half collar which surrounds the medial capsule.

Periodic radiological control of these HO is of utmost significance, assisting in the diagnosis of progression, detention, or regression of the process. Bone scintiscan is also extremely useful in the diagnosis of activity of HO.

5.1.4.5 Treatment and Prognosis

HO is rarely a clinical problem, as most cases are minute or mild. However, in certain instances HO determines severe functional joint impairment and even a sort of extra-articular arthrodesis. Thus, resection of the ossified formations becomes necessary. If excision is required, it should never be performed until bone scintiscan and periodic roentgenographic controls show that the area is no longer producing bone [20, 91], i.e., the process is allowed to completely mature [351, 420]. The hip joint impairment may be diminished by excision of the calcified mass, but this is not the rule.

Prognosis in major HO is to be guarded, and a variable degree of impairment of the hip joint function is to be anticipated.

Fig. 5.14. **a** Posterior dislocation of left hip in a 15-year-old girl, who was struck by an automobile. ▷ Closed reduction achieved within 6 h. **b, c** Condition 25 years later: traumatic arthritis has developed, with narrowing of the medial joint space. The superior joint space, though diminished, is preserved. The patient complains of hip and thigh pain after long walks. There is mild limitation of internal rotation

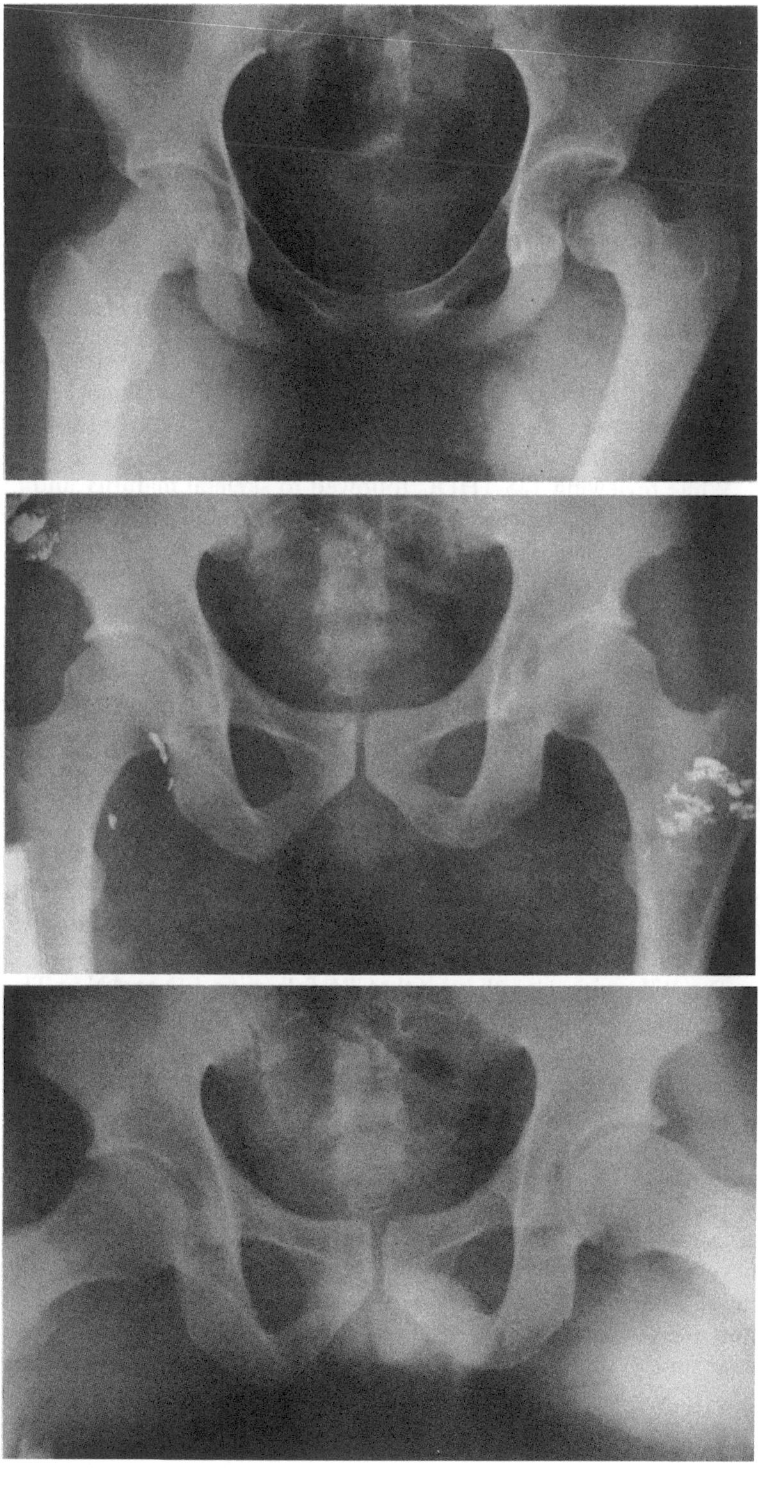

a b c

5.1.5 *Traumatic Arthritis*

Little is known about the incidence and severity of traumatic arthritis (TA) following THDC due to the small number of cases adequately followed during long periods.

The results of simple dislocations in children have usually been considered to be uniformly good, leaving a small number of cases with guarded prognosis for those infrequent severe FD and those cases undergoing AN. Morton said that "it seems likely that since fractures are uncommon in association with hip dislocations in childhood, and since AN occurs in less than 10% of cases, TA can also be said to be uncommon as a complication of THDC." [326]

However, Epstein found, among 51 THDC with long term follow-up, an incidence of AN reaching 6% of the cases, and of TA reaching 12%. TA occurred in three dislocations with or without minor fracture and in three FD. TA following AN were excluded from these cases [146].

While reviewing 145 THDC followed to skeletal maturity and thereafter, with follow-up ranging between 3 and 31 years (mean 11 years), 50 patients - dislocations with associated separation of the capital femoral epiphysis excluded - displayed an abnormal result [29]. Among these 50 patients, there were 26 AN, with or without TA, and 24 TA not secondary to AN. The incidence of TA was obviously higher after FD, but in simple dislocations it was also significant, and this incidence increased with the length of follow-up.

Certain facts emerge from the analysis of this information. First, follow-up after THDC should be prolonged as much as possible in order to draw more freely conclusions about the incidence and characteristics of degenerative arthritis, as also stated by others [163, 351, 413]. Second, the incidence of TA following THDC is high, much higher than usually considered, not only after FD or AN, but also even after adequately treated simple dislocations not developing AN. A further conclusion might be that, although significant, the incidence of TA in THDC is lower than in THDA due to the significantly higher frequency of FD and severe causative trauma in adults, as also found by others [11, 146, 495].

The WS review also showed that TA following FD or AN in THDC may be of early apparition, occurring within a few years, although a high percentage of instances occur in the second or third decades of life. Meanwhile, TA secondary to anterior and type 1 posterior dislocations usually appear later, in mid-adult ages or afterwards.

The major factors leading to a predisposition toward the development of TA following THDC are, as previously discussed: FD causes morphological changes at the joint, which lead to degenerative joint disease, especially if the superior dome of the acetabulum is damaged, with disturbance of the relationship of this part of the socket to the head of the femur [256]. AN, due to the resultant joint incongruity, may lead to TA in a significant percentage of cases [27]. The third etiologic factor, even in simple dislocations, is severe trauma, causing chondral lesions, which if overlooked at the time of injury will be responsible for the development of TA (Fig. 5.14).

5.1.5.1 Clinical and Radiological Signs

The pathoanatomy and the clinical radiological signs of TA following THDC will not be described in this book. These are similar to those seen for other forms of TA, and are described with excellence elsewhere. I shall only add that narrowing of the cartilaginous hip space and spur formation, together with progressive deformity of the femoral head and acetabulum, do not mean significant joint impairment in all instances. In a number of these patients, functional results, in spite of the radiological findings, are not so bad, and an acceptable life without precocious surgery is possible. Some patients with TA in these instances are satisfied with their results during prolonged periods, even though there may be some discomfort. Nevertheless, there are other cases in which reconstructive hip surgery needs to be planned and performed due to the significant impairment caused by TA.

5.1.5.2 Treatment

The management of TA following THDC, having developed to a significant extent, has been previously analyzed by several authorities, but it is still a topic of profound discussion.

When surgical treatment is required, the first consideration should be that we are dealing with young patients. The orthopedic surgeon will have to especially rely on osteotomies, arthroplasties, or even on arthrodesis. Total hip replacement should not be performed in these young patients, at least in the majority of cases. The details of these procedures, however, as well as their requirements, cannot be discussed within the scope of this book.

I agree with Kenwright [256] that prevention of the development of TA is the main fact to concentrate on, by means of preventing AN by early reduction of the dislocation and by early reduction and fixation of surgical FD. Whenever AN develops and when changes follow FD, reconstitution of the acetabulum and of the relationship between femoral head and acetabulum should be performed as soon as possible and as much as possible, in order to attempt to limit the consequence of TA. This is another reason to perform a routine clinical and radiological periodic control of these patients, not only up to skeletal maturity, but also during their adult lives.

5.2 Prognosis

Hip joint behavior after THDC is still an object of discussion, with conflicting opinions about factors influencing the outcome and the true incidence of unsatisfactory results. This is due to the small number of cases usually reported, to the heterogeneity of documentation and evaluating criteria in some multicentric studies, and to the usually too brief follow-up in previous series [21, 172, 236, 258, 369, 370, 376, 420].

Undoubtedly, the analysis of collected cases with adequate documentation and with long-term follow-up to at least skeletal maturity seems a useful source of information to provide satisfactory knowledge of the outcome of this injury in children, and of the contributing factors. Seldom has this facet of investigation been performed. Donaldson et al. presented it in a series of 44 collected cases [370]. I performed a statistical evaluation in 1983; 143 cases were analyzed, including two bilateral cases, thus constituting 145 "hips" to investigate [29]. Further cases have been collected since then, reaching 157 hips, but their inclusion did not modify our previous findings. For the purpose of these studies, a hip was considered abnormal if there was pain, limited motion, shortening of the limb, limp, or if there were radiographical abnormalities [370].

5.2.1 Factors of Influence

Several theoretically potential influencing factors were evaluated, as follows: age, sex, severity of injury, variety of dislocation, type of dislocation, interval before reduction, reduction procedure, postreduction immobilization, interval before weight-bearing, and recurrent dislocation.

The conclusions of the statistical analysis [29] are as follows:

Age of the Patient. There is a sort of protection in children under 6 years of age, and a higher incidence of complications and abnormal results in children older than 10 years.

Severity of the causative Trauma. There is an increasing incidence of abnormal results with increasing severity of trauma.

Type of Dislocation. There is a significant increase in abnormal results in FD.

Interval Before Reduction. Reduction delayed until after 24 h, and even after 4 hours, significantly increases the incidence of abnormal results.

As shown statistically, these four factors influence the incidence of abnormal results.

The influence of open reduction procedures on the development of abnormal results has not been definitively assessed, as statistics are not significant in their definition of the problem. Open reduction as a cause of abnormal results is difficult to evaluate since the procedure itself is an admission of the failure of closed treatment, and is reserved for the difficult or complicated cases [172 a].

The only variable to modify is the interval before reduction. Therapeutic measures should be carried out as an emergency: this has been already emphasized in Sect. 4.3. Postreduction immobilization and the interval before weight-bearing do not appear as influencing factors: guidelines for postreduction management should be determined on the basis of the current concept of dislocation of any other weight-bearing joint.

5.2.2 *Incidence of Normal and Abnormal Results*

Chavatte has written that, although considered with optimism in earlier times, the modern conception about the outcome after THDC has changed to a more guarded prognosis, and this idea is the consequence of a longer follow-up of "modern" collected cases [101]. Although few, there are some investigations on long-term results after THDC which have led to the opinion that this injury is not particularly benign. The incidence of unsatisfactory results has been found to reach 16% to 18% of the cases in some of these series [146, 376], and 30% or more in some others [29, 298a, 370, 420].

The review of the WS showed the incidence of abnormal results to be greater than 30%. However, it is interesting to note that before a probability of determination can be made in a statistical analysis, each category to be investigated should consist of comparable data. If the collected information is evaluated altogether - simple dislocations, FD, dislocations resulting from mild injuries and severe traumas, etc. - comparable data is not being handled, and thus determinations cannot be made. For instance, in anterior and posterior simple dislocations the incidence of abnormal results was 23%, and in simple dislocations and FD reduced within 24 h the incidence of these abnormal results decreased to 18.7%. In addition, in simple dislocations undergoing closed reduction within 24 h, the incidence of traumatic arthritis decreased to 9%, with a high percentage of good and very good results in these instances (Figs. 3.3, 3.4, 3.6, 4.6, 5.15, and 5.16). Epstein also found the incidence of abnormal results in 35 simple posterior dislocations in children with closed reduction within 24 h to be 8.7%, i.e., a similar percentage. Undoubtedly, the severity of the causative trauma also plays its role.

These findings led to my opinion that the incidence of normal and abnormal results following THDC should be considered not on the basis of all THDC conjunctly, but on the basis of certain "groups" of dislocations, i.e., simple dislocations resulting from a moderate injury, in a young child, with closed reduction achieved within a few hours; or posterior dislocations with acetabular fractures type 2 in older children, treated with some delay; as well as all other possible different conditions. It is obvious that these distinct "groups" of influencing factors will lead to different results from one case to the other.

I also feel we should not try to uniformly define prognosis after THDC. Prognosis after this injury depends in each case upon the previously analyzed influencing factors. Whatever the incidence of abnormal results after THDC actually is, it is significant: in the best condition, i.e., in the less severe injuries treated in the most adequate manner, the incidence of abnormal results is 9%, which is undoubtedly a high percentage for a lesion usually considered benign.

This relatively significant incidence of abnormal results is the consequence of: (a) a somewhat high frequency of AN-THDC, ranging between 3% and 15% in simple dislocations, i.e., in the most mild lesions, with a significant incidence of deformities and degenerative joint changes in the adult life of these patients; and (b) an increasing incidence of TA, even in the absence of AN, with longer follow-up; in this regard, our findings are similar to those of Upadhyay and Moulton in their combined series of adults and children [495]. This relatively high incidence of TA in the absence of AN is generally related to joint fractures associated with the disloca-

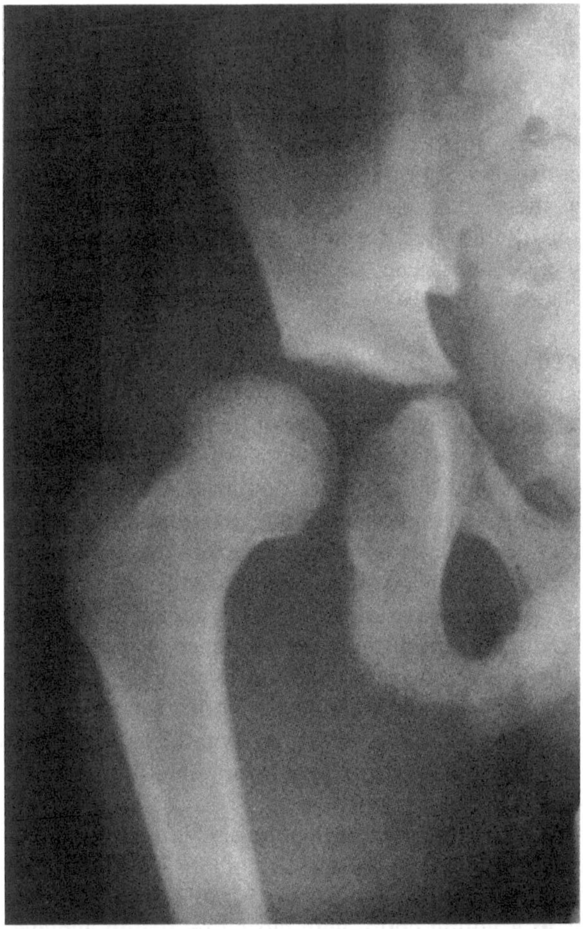
a
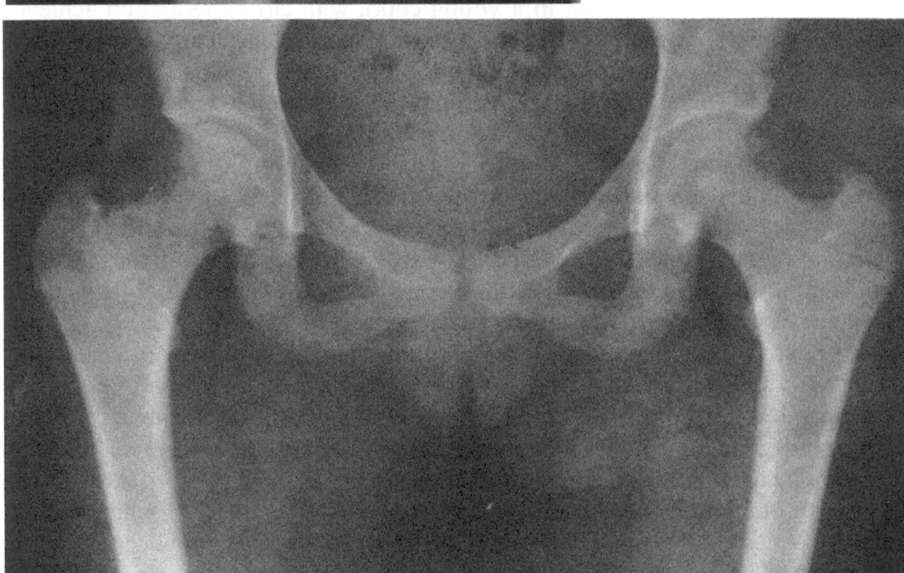
b

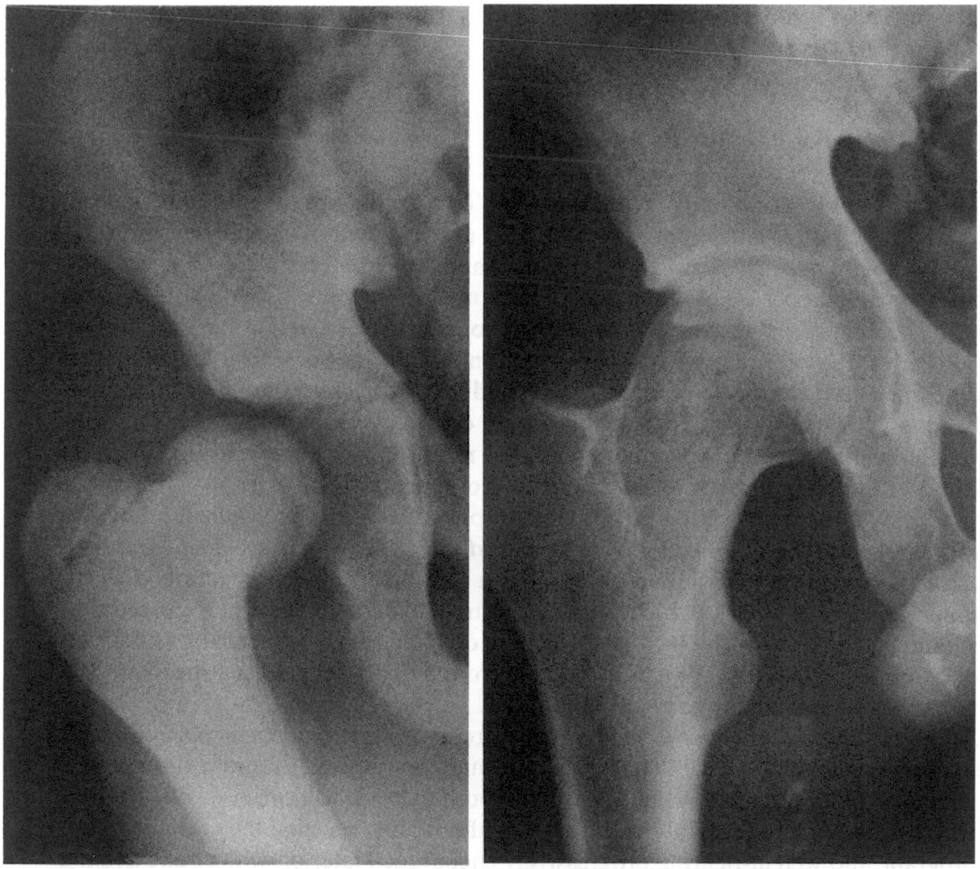

a b

Fig. 5.16. **a** Retroacetabular dislocation of right hip in a 13-year-old boy, who suffered a traffic accident. Closed reduction within 8 h. **b** Condition 35 years later: although there is a small osteophytic formation at the acetabular rim, the joint space is completely preserved and there are no other modifications of the acetabular and femoral head shape. There is no pain or functional limitation

◁ **Fig. 5.15.** **a** Posterior dislocation of right hip in an 11-year-old boy, who was injured while playing football. Closed reduction within 3 h. **b** Condition 17 years later: morphology of the hip is normal, and there is no pain or functional limitation

tion, but also in numerous instances to simple dislocations resulting from severe trauma [29].

5.3 Postreduction Therapeutic Protocol

The analyzed facts about complications and end results following THDC lead to certain conclusions concerning postreduction management of a child with a THD. I suggest for *simple dislocations* with subsequent early closed reduction, i. e., the majority of cases, a period of 4–6 weeks in skin traction or spica cast, to allow for adequate healing of soft tissues, followed by a progessively free weight-bearing. As Ogden states, the presence of synovial irritation should be one of the guidelines to determine the period of protection to the child [351]. The child should begin weight-bearing when pain has subsided, and if pain due to synovial irritation recurs after weight-bearing, it should be interdicted and radiological exams and bone scintiscans performed in order to disclose the development of AN.

For FD, there are certain differences in postreduction management related to the particular type of FD. Confronted with *dislocations with associated acetabular fractures:* type 1 lesions should be treated in the same manner as simple dislocations; types 2, 3, and 4, which are usually treated initially by open procedures, should be managed with prolonged traction, or spica cast when traction is difficult or contraindicated, during periods ranging from 6 to 8 weeks. This appears to be a protocol well accepted by several authorities.

Dislocations with femoral head fracture are exceptions and their postreduction management should be similar to that indicated for types 2, 3, and 4 dislocations with acetabular fracture. Weight-bearing in both these conditions, i. e., dislocations with acetabular and femoral head fractures, should be preceded by a rehabilitation program, and weight-bearing progressively encouraged later on when bone healing and a satisfactory range of joint-motion has been achieved.

Dislocations with separation of the capital femoral epiphysis should be immobilized by cast for a 6- to 8-week period, followed by an adequate rehabilitation program. Permission for weight-bearing should be given depending on the hip-joint condition, and several months may have elapsed until then. *Dislocations with femoral neck fracture* should be managed following a similar protocol.

When a *trochanteric avulsion* has been surgically treated, by means of cerclage wiring, traction or cast treatment should be necessary for 6 weeks and weight-bearing encouraged after 2 further weeks, with progressive active abduction later on.

Periodic evaluating of the involved hip should be performed by clinical, radiological and scintigraphic means, quarterly during the first 2 years, after which clinical and radiological examinations should be performed yearly up to the time of skeletal maturity.

Table 5.1. A total of 170 collected cases of avascular necrosis, following traumatic dislocation of the hip in children

Year	Author	No. of cases	Year	Author	No. of cases
1919	Elmslie	1	1964	Liuboshits et al.	2
1920	Higgins	1	1965	Bonvallet	1
1920	Sundt	2	1965	Fernández	1
1922	Rehbein	1	1965	Titze	2
1923	Fairbank	1	1966	Giglio et al.	1
1931	Bergman	1	1967	Byram et al.	1
1931	Nicolaysen	1	1967	Helal et al.	1
1932	Elsmlie	1	1967	Sanguinetti	1
1932	Pouzet	2	1967	Scialpi et al.	1
1934	Phemister	1	1968	Chapchal	1
1936	Blumensaat	1	1968	Donaldson et al.	2
1937	Cuche	2	1968	De Paoli et al.	1
1938	Funsten et al.	1	1968	Rigault et al.	2
1938	Goldenberg	1	1969	Hipp	6
1938	Paltrinieri	1	1969	Matsubara et al.	2
1939	Birch-Hirschfeld	1	1970	Fina et al.	3
1939	Kleinberg	1	1971	Boitzy	1
1939	Mutschler	1	1971	Lam	1
1940	Watson-Jones	1	1972	Kanan et al.	2
1941	Banks	1	1973	Pearson et al.	1
1942	Bohler	1	1973	Pollen	1
1945	Quist-Hanssen	1	1974	Coleman	1
1947	Urist	1	1974	Hovelius	1
1950	Lezama	1	1974	Rang	2
1951	Paus	1	1974	Robertson et al.	2[a]
1951	Zarotti	1	1974	Schwartz et al.	1
1953	Mau	1	1975	Chotigavanichaya	7
1955	Barbieri	1	1975	Kuner	1
1955	Jensen	1	1976	Labaziewicz	1
1955	Ruiz	1	1976	Macfarlane et al.	2
1955	Scholder	2	1976	Nerubay	1
1956	Picchio	1	1977	Canale et al.	5
1957	Bohler	1	1977	Rogala et al.	1
1958	Jantzen	1	1978	Hidalgos	2
1958	Jonasch	1	1978	Soares	3
1959	Cros	1	1979	Barquet	4
1959	De Wulf	1	1979	Guillaume	2
1959	Peltokallio et al.	2	1979	Lavianos	1
1960	Seewald	1	1979	Weigand et al.	1
1961	Davalli	1	1980	Bunnell et al.	2
1961	Freeman	2	1980	Epstein	3
1961	Glass et al.	13	1980	Germaneau et al.	2
1961	Gouin	1	1980	Mass et al.	1
1961	Haliburton et al.	1	1981	Barquet	1
1961	Piggot	1	1981	Canale	2[b]
1962	Altav	7	1981	Offierski	1[c]
1962	Funk	2	1983	Fiddian et al.	1
1962	Ruffoni	1	1983	Petrini et al.	3
1962	Ulloa	4	1983	Sinha et al.	4
1963	Ricci et al.	1	1984	Collado et al.	1

[a] Three further cases previously published by Fina et al.
[b] Five further cases previously published in 1977.
[c] Also reports 47% incidence of coxa magna.

6 Unreduced Dislocations

6.1 Introduction

Several chronological criteria have been applied when defining late unreduced THD, i.e., 72 h [175], 1 week [354], 3 weeks [163], etc. The criteria used in this book are based on the fact that when reduction of the dislocation is delayed more than 24 h, the incidence of AN shows an extremely high rise, and this significantly affects the outcome. Thus, late unreduced THD is defined as a hip remaining dislocated for more than 24 h.

Fortunately, most THDC are reduced within the initial few hours nowadays. However, late unreduced THDC still occur, offering great difficulties in management and usually presenting an unsatisfactory prognosis. The reason for the occurrence of a late unreduced THD is nearly always the same: except for certain exceptional cases of children who remain at home because their parents do not seek medical advice, unreduced dislocations are the consequence of diagnostic failures of the attending orthopedic surgeon.

6.2 Etiologic Circumstances

Late unreduced THDC are usually the result of severe accidents in which coma, multiple injuries, fracture of the same femur or tibia, or injuries to the contralateral hip distract the attention from the dislocated hip [21, 25, 57, 114, 175, 218, 233, 367, 401, 509]. Other etiologic circumstances of this condition in children are: (a) THD resulting from trivial trauma, with mild functional symptoms and mild vicious attitude of the limb, especially in certain posterior dislocations; thus, dislocation may be overlooked, diagnosis being a simple contusion and X-rays not being performed; and (b) retroacetabular dislocation, due to reasons discussed previously in this book.

6.3 Pathoanatomy

There is adequate information on the pathoanatomy of late unreduced THDC from numerous reported cases of open procedures performed in patients in this age group, especially in the initial decades of this century [16, 77, 105, 124, 184, 203, 209, 219, 302, 306, 524].

After 3 or 4 weeks have elapsed, the acetabular socket is progressively filled with connective tissue, which firmly sticks to the bottom of the socket and becomes more compact. The femoral head, still intact, is surrounded by a thick layer of fibrous tissue.

Later on, the fibroconnective tissue filling the acetabulum may ossify, and therefore the depth of the socket diminishes. The cavity may even disappear in some months, making attempts at reduction very difficult. The fibrous peel surrounding the femoral head grows thicker, with the surface of the head being covered by fibrocartilaginous tissue. A neo-joint is conformed, which may allow a certain degree of mobility.

However, lesions progress, leading to ankylosis, which is initially of the fibrous type. As time passes, ossification takes place and the femoral head is so fixed, that it may be impossible to free it even by surgery. The femoral head remains without alteration for longer periods than the acetabulum - for some 2 to 3 months the articular cartilage is usually intact [399]. Thereafter, there is progressive cartilaginous degeneration, and in addition, as a result of osteoporosis, the femoral head becomes smooth and may even partially resorb; the femoral neck shortens and appears in the line of the femoral shaft, and the trochanters may eventually fix to the acetabulum. Shortening of muscles, tendons, nerves, and vessels becomes increasingly greater. This is another aspect to consider, not only because shortening of muscles and tendons contributes to making reduction extremely difficult, but also because acute reduction may injure nerves and vessels, with severe sequela resulting.

Therefore, a late unreduced dislocation will be extremely difficult to reduce weeks or months after the injury, even by open procedures. In case reduction is achieved, definitive sequela of varying degrees will occur at the joint, frequently associated with AN of the PFE.

6.4 Clinical and Radiological Features

Disability in these "neglected" dislocations is often significant, and children are brought in for medical treatment because of limp and pain of variable severity. However, disability in children may possibly be mild or moderate, and this for long periods [184, 302]; there appears to be something like a "tolerance" for these changes in some children.

The physical examination shows the typical attitude of the lower limb of a hip dislocation, stiffness of the hip joint, and the child walks badly, with a shortened limb and compensatory attitudes at the spine and pelvis. These symptoms and signs increase in severity with time, due to degenerative changes occurring at the femoral head, acetabulum, pelvis, and spine. There is increasing disability, and active treatment is necessary.

6.5 Treatment

Treatment of late unreduced THDC is challenging, and there is no general agreement on a management protocol.

Maneuvers attempting closed reduction are efficient in most cases in the initial few days, but the incidence of poor results in these instances is extremely high due to the development of AN. Statistically, THD is irreducible by closed maneuvers after 2-3 weeks following the dislocation. This procedure also presents a high risk of fracture of the femur upon manipulation in late cases, and otherwise is not indicated in FD, except for those belonging to type 1 dislocation with acetabular fracture.

Heavy skeletal traction for few days and reduction of the dislocation by abducting the leg has been successful in several simple posterior dislocations and is recommended in the literature [38, 61, 67, 98, 202, 203, 354, 400]. The fibrous tissue surrounding the dislocated hip can be stretched by continuous heavy traction; the femur is descended and may be placed in front of the acetabulum. Skeletal traction of up to 18 kg has been applied by Gupta and Shravat [203]; when the femoral head is in front of the acetabulum or even below its level, the limb is gradually abducted in posterior dislocations and traction progressively relaxed. The femoral head is thus reduced into the acetabulum. It should be added that traction should be performed under sedation, and that after reduction is accomplished traction is maintained for another 2-3 weeks. By using this procedure soft tissues are more relaxed, less pressure is exerted on the articular cartilage, and no manipulative reduction is required [203]. Therefore, the incidence of AN is significantly diminished as compared with closed maneuvers for the unreduced dislocations. Gupta and Shravat recommend this method for the initial 10 weeks [203], but Oni et al. have reported satisfactory results even in dislocations neglected for longer periods [354].

Open reduction following heavy traction is necessary to remove acetabular debris and scar tissue, which avoids concentric reduction. Garrett et al. consider that in young patients with type 2 or 3 FD of less than 3 months duration, open reduction with removal of bone fragments and internal fixation of the fracture may be recommended [175]. However, this is a difficult procedure and results are dissappointing in a high number of instances.

Some authors prefer to leave the head dislocated, especially in cases older than 3 months, recommending a *corrective osteotomy,* to improve the pathologic position of the limb, performed at the trochanteric or subtrochanteric level [46, 52, 63, 202, 209, 283]. The osteotomy would ameliorate the gait and pelvic stability. Hamada has stated that "corrective osteotomy of the femur at the trochanteric region is the simplest corrective operation" [209]. However, another clinical state indicating this operation would be a relatively pain-free hip with an acceptable range of joint flexion. This procedure has several disadvantages, i.e., limb length inequality is not adequately corrected, the pelvis and spine are surcharged, and total hip replacement will be more or less impossible to perform in the future.

Reduction arthrodesis has also been used and recommended for long-standing old dislocations [98, 104, 281, 328, 360, 502, 517], in a search for a stable and painless hip which, though rigid, may permit a somewhat acceptable solution for these patients. In addition, it permits a total hip replacement in the future. However, injuries or previous disabling affections at the spine, the ipsilateral knee, and the controlateral hip contraindicate reduction arthrodesis of the hip [175].

Cup arthroplasty is seldom performed nowadays, whereas *total hip replacement* should not be performed in children.

In spite of the controversial recommendations in the previous literature, certain guidelines for management of unreduced THDC may be suggested. Although closed maneuvers are advocated in the initial few days after the dislocation, a significant incidence of complicating AN must be anticipated.

For unreduced THDC of less than 3 months duration, the procedure described by Gupta and Shravat [203], consisting of heavy skeletal traction and subsequent abduction (for posterior dislocations), seems to be a formal requirement. Possibly adduction should be added for anterior cases. Undoubtedly this method is mostly restricted to simple dislocations, but most of these cases in children are not associated with joint fractures. An example is shown in Fig. 6.1.

Whenever this procedure fails, and also in very old cases, in FD types 2, 3, and 4, and in dislocations with associated fractures of the proximal femur, open reduction of the dislocation or reduction arthrodesis should be performed in order to prepare a way for a future total hip replacement, which later will give these patients a painless, efficient functioning of their hip joint, when circumstances require this solution in their adult lives.

And last but not least, I feel that the treatment of unreduced dislocations is not the real problem for which one must find a solution. If orthopedic surgeons learn to diagnose and to treat THDC early and adequately, the extremely severe and disagreeable condition of an old neglected THD will undoubtedly disappear.

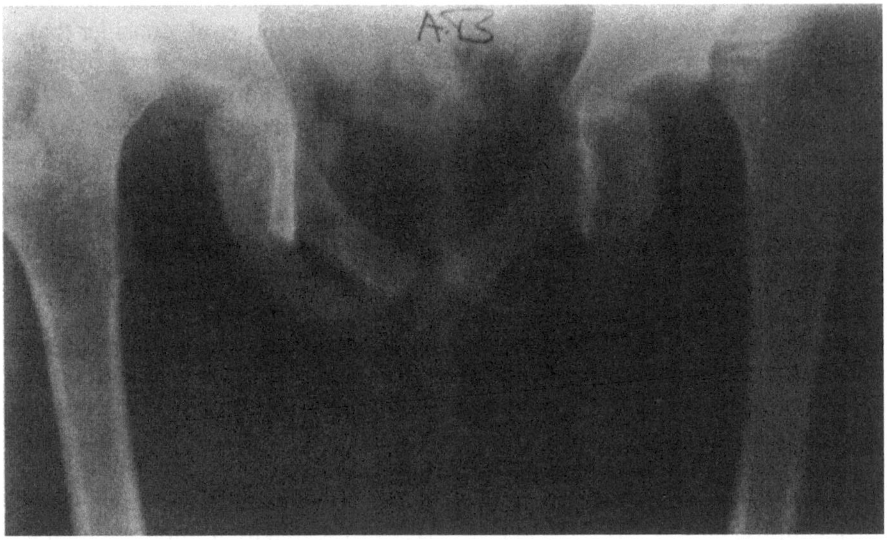

a

Fig. 6.1. **a** X-ray taken on the day of the injury of a 5-year-old girl who was riding seated on a coaster sled – "no fractures" reported. The bilateral dislocations are apparent. **b** X-ray taken at the time of hospitalization 5 weeks after dislocation. Note the marked subchondral osteoporosis of both femoral heads. Heavy skeletal traction was performed, and reduction was noted on the 5th day of traction. **c** Radiological condition 18 months following reduction. The patient's examination was considered normal. (From Bunnell and Webster [61])

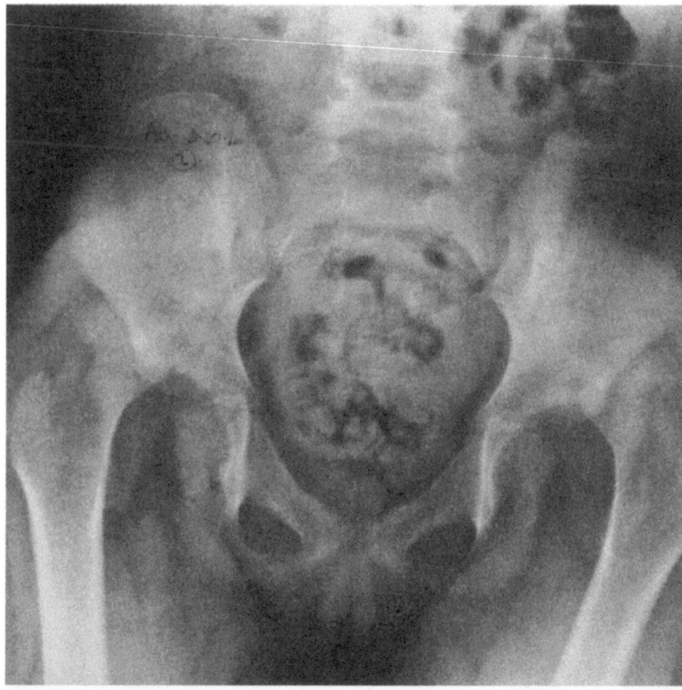
b

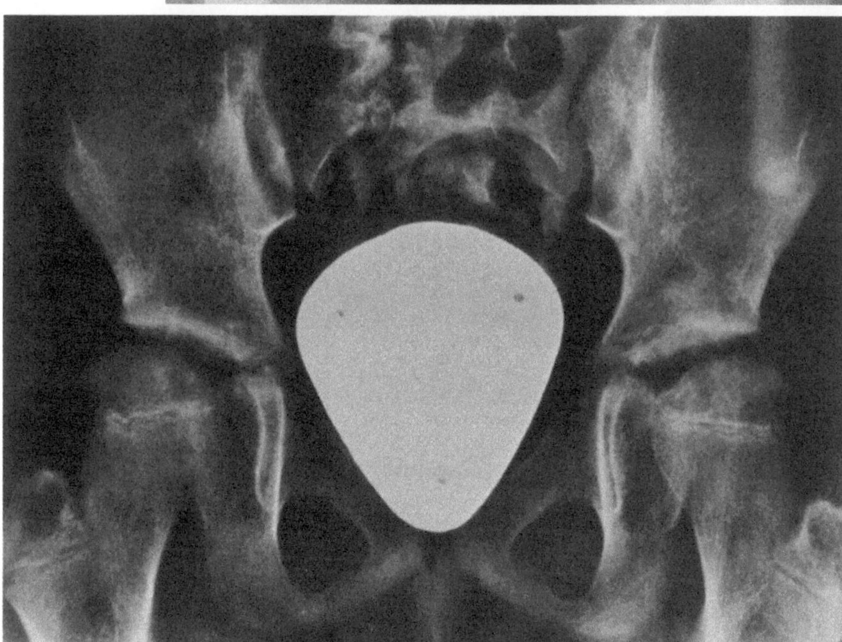
c

References

1. Abad Rico J: Personal communication
2. Abad Rico J, Barquet A (1982) Luxatio erecta of the hip. Arch Orthop Traumat Surg 99: 277-279
3. Alcívar E (1946) Obstetrical dislocation of the hip associated with fracture of the femur. J Bone Joint Surg 28: 838-841
4. Alho A (1980) Injuries in the femoral axis. Int Orthop 3: 271-279
5. Allis O (1896) An inquiry into the difficulties encountered in the reduction of dislocations of the hip. Dornan, Philadelphia
6. Alms O (1961) Fracture mechanics. J Bone Joint Surg [Br] 43: 162-166
7. Altav H (1962) Erfahrungen mit der kindlichen traumatischen Hüftluxation in der Türkei. Verh Dtsch Orthop Ges 50: 308
8. Amihoood S (1974) Posterior dislocation of the hip. S Afr Med J 48: 1029-1032
9. Andreini G (1956) La lussazione traumatica dell'anca. Ortop Traumat 24: 815-835
10. Arancio A, Galimberti G (1968) La lussazione traumatica dell'anca nei bambini. Atti SERTOT 18: 51-54
11. Armstrong J (1948) Traumatic dislocation of the hip joint. J Bone Joint Surg [Br] 30: 430-455
12. Aufranc O, Jones W, Harris H (1964) Recurrent traumatic dislocation of the hip in a child. JAMA 190: 291-294
13. Ayrolo A (1955) Luxación traumática de cadera en un niño de 9 años. Bol Trab Soc Arg Ortop Traumatol, Sesión del 19 de Julio de 1955

13a. Azouz E (1983) Apparent or true neonatal dislocation? Radiologic differential diagnosis. Can Med Assoc J 129: 595-597

14. Bado J: personal communication
15. Bairov G (1952) Case of open dislocation of the hip in a child. Vestn Khir 72: 68-69
16. Bajardi D (1900) Riduzione cruenta di lussazione ileo-pettinea del femore sinistro. Arch Ortop 17: 145-162
17. Banks S (1941) Aseptic necrosis of the femoral head following traumatic dislocation of the hip. J Bone Joint Surg 23: 753-781
18. Barbieri M (1955) Distacco-lussazione dell'epifisi femorale prossimale. Chir Organi Mov 41: 338-340
19. Barcat J, Testas P (1958) A propos des luxations traumatiques récentes de la hanche chez l'enfant. Mém Acad Chir 84: 659-663
20. Barquet A (1979) Luxación traumática de la cadera en la infancia. Monograph, Faculty of Medicine, Montevideo
21. Barquet A (1979) Traumatic hip dislocation in childhood. Acta Orthop Scand 50: 549-553
22. Barquet A (1980) Luxations traumatiques irréductibles de la hanche chez l'enfant. Lyon Chir 76: 329-330
23. Barquet A (1980) Recurrent traumatic dislocation of the hip in childhood. J Trauma 20: 1003-1006
24. Barquet A (1981) Luxación traumática retroacetabular de la cadera. Acta Ortop Latinoam 8: 25-27
25. Barquet A (1981) Traumatic hip dislocation with fracture of the ipsilateral femoral shaft in childhood. Arch Orthop Trauma Surg 98: 69-72
26. Barquet A (1982) Avascular necrosis following traumatic hip dislocation in childhood. Acta Orthop Scand 53: 809-813

27. Barquet A (1982) Natural history of avascular necrosis following traumatic hip dislocation in childhood. Acta Orthop Scand 53: 815–820
28. Barquet A (1982) Traumatic anterior dislocation of the hip in childhood. Injury 13: 435–440
29. Barquet A (in press) Los resultados alejados de la luxación traumática de la cadera en la infancia. Acta Ortop Latinoam
30. Barquet A, Leborgne J (in press) La tomografia computada en las luxo-fracturas de cadera. Rev Soc Ortop Traum Urug
30a. Barquet A, Fernández A, León H (1985) Simultaneous ipsilateral trochanteric and femoral shaft fracture. Acta Orthop Scand 56: 36–39
31. Barquet A, Vécsei V (1984) Traumatic dislocation of the hip with separation of the proximal femoral epiphysis. Arch Orthop Trauma Surg 103: 219–223
32. Bartels M (1874) Traumtische Luxationen. Arch Klin Chir 16: 636–654
33. Bassetta G (1923) Contributo alla casistica della lussazione traumatica dell'anca nell'infanzia. Arch Ortop 38: 591–592
34. Beck E (1979) Therapie der Hüftluxationen. Unfallheilkunde 140: 221–232
35. Bell C (1896) Old traumatic dislocation of the hip; operation; recovery. Lancet 2: 1059
36. Benecke H (1970) Das Kombinationstrauma im Kindesalter. Beitr Orthop Traumatol 17: 253–256
37. Berendes J (1886) Ueber die Luxatio obturatoria. Thesis, Würzburg
38. Bergoin M, Menguy P, Lizarraga L, Carcassonne M (1968) Luxation traumatique "ancienne" de la hanche chez une fillette de 21 mois. Marseille Chir 20: 108–113
39. Bernhang A (1970) Simultanenous bilateral traumatic dislocation of the hip in a child. J Bone Joint Surg [Am] 52: 365–366
40. Bigelow H (1869) Mechanism of dislocation and fracture of the hip with the reduction of the dislocations by the flexion method. Lea and Febiger, Philadelphia
41. Bigelow H (1878) Iliac dislocation in a seven year-old boy reduced after five months. Lancet 1: 86
42. Bijlsma K (1974) Traumatic dislocation of the hip in children (in Dutch). Ned T Geneesk 118: 1586–1589
43. Birch-Hirschfeld A (1939) Die Schenkelkopfnekrose des Jugendlichen nach traumatischer Hüftluxation und ihre Bedeutung für die Begutachtung. Monatsschr Unfallheilkd 46: 241–245
44. Birkett J (1869) Description of a dislocation of the head of the femur complicated with its fracture. Med Chir Trans 52: 133–134
45. Blanco L, Echegaray E (1942) Luxación traumática de la cadera en el niño. Rev Med Cienc Afines 4: 678–680
46. Blount W (1955) Fractures in children. Williams and Wilkins, Baltimore
47. Bloxham J (1833) Dislocation of the hip with fracture of the thigh. London Med Gaz 12: 702–703
48. Blumensaat C (1936) Über sekundäre Schenkelkopfnekrosen nach traumatischer Hüftgelenksverrenkung. Arch Klin Chir 185: 720–752
49. Body J (1969) Luxation récidivante de la hanche chez un garçon. Rev Chir Orthop 55: 65–68
50. Boehnke E (1913) Beitrag zur traumatischen Hüftgelenksluxation bei Kindern. Arch Klin Chir 102: 1077–1091
51. Bohler J (1957) Die sogenannten Schenkelkopfnekrosen nach traumatischen Hüftverrenkungen. Wiederherstellungschir-Traumatol 4: 75–108
52. Bohler L (1938) Technik der Knochenbruchbehandlung. Maudrich, Vienna
53. Boitzy A (1971) A fracture du col de fémur chez l'enfant et l'adolescent. Masson, Paris
54. Bonnemaison M, Henderson E (1968) Traumatic anterior dislocation of the hip with acute common femoral occlusion in a child. J Bone Joint Surg [Am] 50: 753–756
55. Bonvallet J (1965) Sur un cas exceptionnel de luxation traumatique de la hanche chez l'enfant, associée à un décollement épiphysaire complet et à une fracture du noyau céphalique. Rev Chir Orthop 51: 723–728
56. Borchard H (1902) Ein Beitrag zu der Luxatio supra pubica kompliziert durch Fractur des Trochanter major und eine Hernie praevascularis. Dtsch Z Chir 66: 572–578
57. Brav E (1962) Traumatic dislocation of the hip. J Bone Joint Surg [Am] 44: 1115–1134
58. Brug E, Ziegelmuller F (1974) Die traumatische Hüftgelenksluxation im Kindesalter. Münch Med Wochenschr 116: 315–320

59. Brunner G (1953) Über die Hüftgelenksverrenkung unter besonderer Berücksichtigung der seltenen Luxatio coxae ventralis pubica. Monatsschr Unfallheilkd 56: 246-248
60. Bucholz R, Ogden J (1978) Patterns of ischemic necrosis of the proximal femur in nonoperatively treated congenital hip disease. In: The hip. Mosby, St. Louis
61. Bunnell W, Webster D (1980) Late reduction of bilateral traumatic hip dislocations in a child. Clin Orthop 147: 160-163
62. Burci E (1895) Notizie cliniche e ricerche sugli infermi operate in quattro semestri si servizio chirurgico. N. Spitale di Pisa, Pisa
63. Byram G, Wickstrom J (1967) Traumatic dislocation of the hip in children. South Med J 60: 805-810
64. Caamaño A (1941) Luxaciones traumáticas de la cadera en el niño. Semana Méd 48: 1450-1457
65. Cagnoli H (1952) Les fractures articulaires de la hanche (à l'exception du col du fémur). Rev Orthop 38: 494-512
66. Cagnoli H (1968) Fracturas del cotilo. In: Lesiones traumáticas de pelvis. Oficina del Libro-AEM, Montevideo
67. Calderon C (1950) Desprendimiento y luxación traumática de la epífisis superior del fémur. Cir Ap Locom 7: 393-397
68. Campailla E (1967) La lussazione traumatica d'anca nell'infanzia. Clin Orthop 19: 623-628
69. Campbell W (1927) Perineal dislocation of the hip with avulsion of the greater tuberosity. JAMA 78: 1115-1116
70. Canale S (1981) Traumatic dislocations and fracture-dislocations of the hip in children. In: Salvatti EA (ed) The hip. Mosby, St. Louis
71. Canale S, Bourland W (1977) Fractures of the neck and intertrochanteric region of the femur in children. J Bone Joint Surg [Am] 59: 431-443
72. Canale S, Manugian A (1979) Irreducible traumatic dislocations of the hip. J Bone Joint Surg [Am] 61: 7-14
73. Carlioz H, Michelutti D (1982) Traumatismes du bassin et de la hanche chez l'enfant. Ann Chir 36: 50-56
74. Carpi R (1960) Sulla lussazione traumatica dell'anca nell'infanzia. Min Ortop 11: 297-298
75. Cartron P (1925) Contribution a l'étude des luxations traumatiques obturatrices de la hanche. Thesis, Bordeaux
76. Cataldi G, Riella J: personal communication
77. Catoir J (1898/1899) Méthode de douceur dans la réduction des luxations de la hanche en arriere. Thesis, Paris
77a. Cauchoix J, Ramadier J (1949) Sur le traitement des luxations traumatiques anciennes de la hanche. Rev Chir Orthop 35: 548-551
78. Ciliani H: personal communication
79. Clark A (1896) A case of dislocation of the hip-joint in a child of four years. Br Med J 6: 786
80. Clarke H (1928) Traumatic dislocation of the hip-joint in a child. Br J Surg 16: 690-692
81. Clawson D, Melcher P (1975) Fractures and dislocations of the hip. In: Rockwood C, Green D (eds) Fractures. Lippincott, Philadelphia
82. Coello A, Llanos L, Avellanosa J, González C, Corbatón V, Núñez-Samper M (1978) Luxación traumática de la cadera en el niño. Rev Ortop Traum 22 IB: 65-80
83. Cofre Cerda A (1948) Consideraciones sobre algunas afecciones de la cadera en el niño. Arch Hosp Niñ Río 16: 119-123
84. Coimbra A (1938) Luxaçoes traumaticas da coxofemural na criança. Arq Bras Cir Ortop 6: 149-158
85. Coleman S (1974) Aseptic necrosis of bone due to trauma. Orthop Clin North Am 5: 819-832
86. Collado J, Vivas J, Sesma P (1984) Asociación de luxación posterior de cadera y epifisiolisis traumática femoral superior. Rev Ortop Traum 28 IB: 233-236
87. Connolly J (1981) De Palma's The management of fractures and dislocations. Saunders, Philadelphia
88. Cooke W (1864) Dislocation of head of femur into the thyroid foramen, with fracture of the upper part of the shaft; reduction; perfect recovery. Lancet 1: 37-38
89. Cooper A (1823) A treatise on dislocations and on fractures of the joints. Longman-Hurst, London

90. Cormier J, Genin J (1964) Les lésions artérielles des luxations de la hanche. Mem Acad Chir 90: 429-432
91. Craig C (1980) Hip injuries in children and adolescents. Orthop Clin North Am 11: 753-754
92. Crock H (1965) A revision of the anatomy of the arteries supplying the upper end of the human femur. J Anat 99: 77-88
93. Crock H, Dickens D (1984) The blood supply of the upper end of the human femur, including observations on the venous drainage of the femoral head. In: Tronzo R (ed) Surgery of the hip joint. Springer, Berlin Heidelberg New York Tokyo
94. Cros A (1959) Osteochondrosis of the upper femoral epiphysis following traumatic dislocation of the hip joint. J Bone Joint Surg [Am] 41: 1335-1338
95. Cuche M (1936/1937) Résultats éloignés de la réduction précoce des luxations traumatiques de la hanche. Thesis, Lyon
96. Curtillet J, Lombarg P (1911) Luxation traumatique de la hanche chez une petite fille de trois ans et demi; réduction non sanglante quatre-vingt jours après l'accident. Rev Orthop 5: 477-478
97. Chakraborti S, Miller I (1975) Dislocation of the hip associated with fracture of the femoral head. Injury 7: 134-136
98. Chapchal G (1968) Cirugía ortopédica y traumatológica de la cadera. Científico Médica, Barcelona
99. Charry V (1936) Luxation traumatique invétérée de la hanche chez un enfant de sept ans et demi réduite par voie sanglante deux mois après l'accident. Rev Orthop 23: 147-152
100. Charry V (1937) Résultat éloigné d'une luxation traumatique de la hanche datant de deux mois et réduite par voie sanglante chez un enfant. Bull Mém Soc Chir 29: 160-163
101. Chavatte J (1968) Luxations traumatiques de la hanche chez l'enfant. Thèse Lyon
102. Chigot P: quoted by Barcat J, Testas P (Reference 19)
103. Chigot P, Esteve P (1957) Traumatologie infantile. Expansion Scientifique, Paris
104. Chotigavanichaya C (1975) Traumatic dislocation of the hip joint in childhood. J Med Assoc Thai 58: 329-336
105. Choyce C (1924) Traumatic dislocation of the hip in childhood and relation of trauma to pseudo-coxalgia: analysis of 59 cases published up to January 1924. Br J Surg 12: 52-59
106. Chung S (1976) The arterial supply of the developing proximal end of the human femur. J Bone Joint Surg [Am] 58: 961-970
107. Chung S (1981) Hip disorders in infants and children. Lea and Febiger, Philadelphia
108. Dall D, Macnab I, Gross A (1970) Recurrent anterior dislocation of the hip. J Bone Joint Surg [Am] 52: 574-576
109. Dambrin L, Dambrin P (1937) Luxation rétro-cotyloïdienne pure traumatique de la hanche; son diagnostique radiologique. Rev Orthop 24: 249-250
110. Dameron T (1959) Bucket-handle tear of acetabular labrum accompanying posterior dislocation of the hip. J Bone Joint Surg [Am] 41: 131-134
111. Davalli C (1961) Due casi di lussazione traumatica dell'anca nel bambino. Arch CTO INAIL 1: 243-361
112. Decoulx J, Duquennoy A, Spy E (1971) L'origine radiculaire des paralysies sciatiques par luxation-fracture de la hanche. Rev Chir Orthop 57: 335-373
113. De Guidi G, Grassi E, Nicosia U (1967) La lussazione traumatica dell'anca nell'infanzia. Minerva Pediatr 19: 129-136
114. Dehne E, Immermann E (1951) Dislocation of the hip combined with fracture of the shaft of the femur on the same side. J Bone Joint Surg [Am] 33: 731-745
115. Delagarde P (1866) Resection of the head of the femur for unreduced dislocation into the ischiatic notch. St. Barthol Hosp Rec 2: 183-184
116. DeLee J, Evans J, Thomas J (1980) Anterior dislocation of the hip and associated femoral head fractures. J Bone Joint Surg [Am] 62: 960-964
117. Denettieres J (1890) Causes des luxations irréductibles de la hanche. Thèse Paris
118. De Pena P, Gaudiano J, Berriolo A, Suero C, Touya E (1984) Comparación entre centellografía ósea y de médula ósea en diagnóstico de isquemia de epífisis femoral. 4th Cong Bras Biol Med Nuclear, P. Alegre, p 53
119. De Wulf A, van Vynckt C (1950) Luxation ouverte de la hanche chez un jeune garçon polytraumatise. Acta Orthop Belg 16: 514-519

120. De Wulf A (1959) Suites lointaines d'une luxation ouverte de la hanche chez un jeune garçon de 14 ans. Acta Orthop Belg 25: 671-675
121. Dialer S (1965) Seltene Form einer Hüftverrenkung beim Jugendlichen. Klin Med 21: 221-223
122. Dingley A, Denham R (1964) Pubic dislocation of the hip. J Bone Joint Surg [Am] 46: 865-867
123. Dixson C (1889) Dislocation on to the dorsum ilii in a child six years old. Lancet 2: 902
124. Doelle O (1921) Beitrag zur traumatischen Hüftgelenksluxation bei Kindern. Arch Klin Chir 118: 703-725
125. Doljnitzkij O (1960) On traumatic dislocation of the hip in children. Ortop Travmatol Protez 21: 74-76
126. Dollinger J (1911) Die veralteten traumatischen Verrenkungen der Schulter, des Ellenbogens und der Hüfte. Ergeb Chir Orthop 3: 83-194
127. Douglas T (1889) Dislocation of the right hip in a boy aged seven years and a half. Lancet 2: 952
128. Doutrelepont H: quoted by Giraud D (Reference 184)
129. Drehmann G (1896) Zur operativen Behandlung irreponibler traumatischer Hüftgelenksluxation. Beitr Klin Chir 17: 775-802
130. Drevermann P (1924) Isolierte Luxation iliaca des Schenkelkopfes bei traumatischer Epiphysenlösung. Dtsch Z Chir 185: 422-426
131. Duahine M, Labelle P, Duchesne R (1976) Traumatic dislocation of the hip in children. J Bone Joint Surg [Br] 48: 138
132. Duncan C, Shim S (1977) Blood supply of the head of the femur in traumatic hip dislocation. Surg Gynecol Obstet 144: 185-191
133. Dupuis R (1855) Luxation ovalaire chez un enfant de 12 ans. Rev Méd-Chir, Bordeaux
134. Durbin F (1959) Avascular necrosis complicating undisplaced fractures of the neck of femur in children. J Bone Joint Surg [Br] 41: 758-762
135. Duriez J (1977) Réflexions à propos de la physiopathologie de l'ostéochondrite de la hanche. Rev Chir Orthop 63: 157-172
136. Duyfjes F (1963) Recurrent dislocation of the hip joint in a boy. J Bone Joint Surg [Br] 45: 432
137. Economu T, Gavrilita N, Nastase N (1958) Formes rares de luxation traumatique de la hanche chez les enfants. Lyon Chir 54: 203-210
138. Ehalt W (1962) Traumatische Hüftluxationen beim Kind. Verh Dtsch Orthop Ges 50: 309
139. Ehtisham S (1976) Traumatic dislocation of hip joint with fracture of shaft of femur on the same side. J Trauma 16: 196-205
140. Eisenberg K, Sheft D, Murray W (1972) Posterior dislocation of the hip producing lumbosacral nerve-root avulsion. J Bone Joint Surg [Am] 54: 1083-1086
141. Ekstrand J, Tkazcuk H (1983) Epifyseolys vid traumatisk hoftledsluxation - en salsynt komplikation. Lakartidningen 80: 1329-1330
142. Elsmlie R (1919) Pseudocoxalgia following traumatic dislocation of the hip in a boy aged four years. J Orthop Surg 1: 109-114
143. Elsmlie R (1932) Traumatic dislocation of the hip in a child aged seven, with subsequent development of coxa plana. Proc R Soc Med 25: 100-101
144. Emmola P, Ando E (1959) Contributo allo studio clinico della lussazione traumatica d'anca nell'infanzia. Atti SOTIMI 4: 377-380
145. Endlich K (1898) Über die blutige Reposition der Luxatio iliaca and obturatoria. Arch Klin Chir 56: 574-590
146. Epstein H (1980) Traumatic dislocation of the hip. Williams and Wilkins, Baltimore
147. Erlacher: quoted by Giraud D (Reference 184)
148. Eteve L: quoted by Henry A, Bayumi M (Reference 221)
149. Evans D, Loyd-Roberts G (1958) Treatment of Legg-Calvé-Perthes' disease. A comparison of in-patient and out-patient treatment. J Bone Joint Surg 40: 182-191
150. Fairbank H (1924) Case of pseudo-coxalgia following traumatic dislocation in a boy. Proc R Soc Med 17: 40
151. Fardon D (1978) Femoral shaft fracture with ipsilateral hip dislocation in a child. JACEP 7: 159-161
152. Farrant (1889) Dislocation on to the dorsum ilii in a child. Lancet 1: 741
153. Fernandes A (1981) Traumatic posterior dislocation of hip joint with a fracture of the head and neck of the femur on same side. Injury 12: 487-490

154. Fernández J: personal communication
155. Fernández Herrera E (1965) Luxación traumática anterior de la cadera en la infancia. Bol Med Hosp Infant Mex 22: 95-99
156. Ferguson A, Howarth M (1935) Coxa magna. JAMA 104: 808-812
157. Fevre M (1958) Chirurgie infantile d'urgence. Masson, Paris
158. Ficat P, Arlet J (1977) Ischemia et nécrose osseusses. Masson, Paris
159. Fiddian N, Grace D (1983) Traumatic dislocation of the hip in adolescence with separation of the capital epiphysis. J Bone Joint Surg [Br] 65: 148-149
160. Fina C, Kelly P (1970) Dislocations of the hip with fractures of the proximal femur. J Trauma 10: 77-87
161. Fineschi G (1958) Die traumatische Hüftverrenkung bei Kindern. Arch Orthop Unfall-Chir 48: 225-236
162. Fischer L, Imbert J (1969) Luxation traumatique de la hanche rétro-cotyloïdiene pure chez l'enfant, sans déplacement en hauteur. Necessité du cliché de profil. Lyon Med 222: 825-826
163. Fischer L, Venouil J, Baulieux J, Vuillard P, Imbert J, Chavatte J (1971) Luxations traumatiques de la hanche chez l'enfant. Cah Med Lyon 47: 3325-3331
164. Flach A, Kudlich H (1962) Schenkelkopfnekrosen nach traumatischen Hüftluxationen und Schenkelhalsfrakturen Jugendlicher. Zentralbl Chir 87: 860-871
165. Floyd A (1984) Traumatic dislocation of the hip in a child. S Afr Med J 65: 935-937
166. Fordyce A (1971) Open reduction of traumatic dislocation of the hip in a child. Br J Surg 58: 705-707
167. Frankovitch K (1983) Coxa magna, femoral overgrowth of operated limb following open reduction of congenital dislocated hip with medial approach. Orthop Trans 7: 568
168. Freeman G (1961) Traumatic dislocation of the hip in children. J Bone Joint Surg [Am] 43: 401-406
169. Fregnani L, Droghetti I (1970) Risultati lontani della lussazione traumatica dell'anca nella giovane etá. Arcisp S. Anna Ferrara 23: 262-271
170. Fries G (1966) Zur Behandlung veralteter traumatischer Hüftluxationen und Luxationsfrakturen im Kindesalter. Arch Orthop Unfall-Chir 59: 229-239
171. Froelich: quoted by Martel F (Reference 306)
172. Funk F (1962) Traumatic dislocation of the hip in children. J Bone Joint Surg [Am] 44: 1135-1145
172a. Funk F: discussion, following Pennsylvannia Orthopaedic Society (Reference 370)
173. Furtak J (1974) Remote results of treatment of traumatic hip joint dislocation. Chir Narzadow Ruchu Ortop Pol 39: 29-34
174. Funsten R, Kinser P, Frankel C (1938) Dashboard dislocation of the hip. J Bone Joint Surg 20: 124-132
175. Garret J, Epstein H, Harris W, Harvey J, Nickel V (1979) Treatment of unreduced traumatic posterior dislocations of the hip. J Bone Joint Surg [Am] 61: 2.6
176. Gartland J: discussion following Funk F (Reference 172)
177. Gartland J, Benner J (1976) Traumatic dislocations in the lower extremity. Orthop Clin North Am 7: 687-692
178. Garvan J (1983) Delayed presentation of posterior fracture dislocation of the hip in a child. Aust NZ J Surg 53: 493-496
179. Gaul R (1973) Recurrent traumatic dislocation of the hip in children. Clin Orthop 90: 107-109
179a. Germaneau J, Vital J, Bucco P, Bechraoui T, Bondonny J (1980) Luxations traumatiques de la hanche de l'enfant de moins de 6 ans. Chir Pédiatr 21: 239-244
180. Gerster: quoted by Drehmann G (Reference 129)
181. Ghormley R, Sullivan R (1953) Traumatic dislocation of the hip. Am J Surg 85: 298-302
182. Giglio H: discussion, following Loray J (Reference 293)
183. Giglio H, Briones O (1964) Luxación traumática inveterada anterior de la cadera. Terceras Jornadas Rioplatenses de Ortopedia y Traumatología, Córdoba
184. Giraud D (1927) Contribution a l'étude de la luxation traumatique de la hanche chez l'enfant. Thesis, Bordeaux
185. Glass A, Powell H (1961) Traumatic dislocation of the hip in children. J Bone Joint Surg [Br] 43: 29-37
186. Glynn P (1932) Two cases of traumatic dislocation of the hip in children. Lancet 2: 1093

187. Goetz A (1934) Traumatic dislocation of the hip (head of the femur) into the scrotum. J Bone Joint Surg 16: 718-720
188. Gogler E (1960) Unfallopfer im Straßenverkehr. Documenta Geigy, Series Chirurgica 5: 77
189. Goldenberg R (1938) Traumatic dislocation of the hip followed by Perthe's disease. J Bone Joint Surg 20: 770-774
190. Gouin J (1961) A propos des luxations traumatiques de la hanche chez l'enfant. Mém Acad Chir 87: 612-615
191. Gregory C (1973) Early complications of dislocations and fracture-dislocations of the hip joint. In: American Academy of Orthopaedic Surgeons - Instructional course lectures, vol 22. Mosby, Saint Louis
192. Griffin P: quoted by Aufranc O, Jones W, Harris W (Reference 12)
193. Grigovich I (1964) Open dislocation of the hip in a child. Vestn Khir Grakov 92: 83
194. Grob M (1957) Lehrbuch der Kinderchirurgie. Georg Thieme, Stuttgart
195. Grobelski M (1957) Die traumatischen Hüftverrenkungen im Kindesalter. Arch Orthop Unfall-Chir 48: 691-697
196. Grundy M, Kumar N (1982) Open anterior dislocation of the hip. Injury 13: 315-316
197. Guersant: quoted by Martel F (Reference 306)
198. Guglielmone O: personal communication
199. Gui L (1957) Fratture e lussazione. Edizione Scientifici Instituto Ortopédico Toscano, Firence
200. Guillaume E: personal communication
201. Gula D (1972) Recurrent traumatic dislocation of the hip in children. J Am Osteopath Assoc 72: 32-39
202. Gupta A, Chaturvedi S (1970) Traumatic dislocation of hip in childhood (incidence and treatment). Ind J Surg 32: 28-35
203. Gupta R, Shravat B (1977) Reduction of neglected traumatic dislocation of the hip by heavy traction. J Bone Joint Surg [Am] 59: 249-251
204. Gupta R, Gupta K, Singhal A (1981) Traumatic posterior dislocation of the hip in children. Int Surg 65: 445-449
205. Guyer B, Levinsohn E (1983) Recurrent anterior dislocation of the hip: case report with arthrographic findings. Skeletal Radiol 10: 262-264
206. Haedke H (1903) Blutige Reposition einer irreponiblen Hüftgelenksluxation. Dtsch Chir 66: 359-363
207. Haines C (1937) Traumatic dislocation of head of femur in child. J Bone Joint Surg 19: 1126-1127
208. Haliburton R, Brockenshire F, Barber J (1961) Avascular necrosis of the femoral capital epiphysis after traumatic dislocation of the hip in children. J Bone Joint Surg [Br] 43: 43-46
209. Hamada G (1957) Unreduced anterior dislocation of the hip. J Bone Joint Surg [Br] 39: 471-476
210. Hamilton F (1866) A practical treatise on fractures and dislocations. Lea, Philadelphia
211. Hammelbo T (1976) Traumatic hip dislocation in childhood. Acta Orthop Scand 47: 546-548
212. Hampson W (1972) Venous obstruction by anterior dislocation of the hip-joint. Injury 4: 69-73
213. Harper M (1982) Traumatic dislocation of the hip with ipsilateral femoral shaft fracture: a method of treatment. Injury 13: 391-394
214. Harris G (1924) An unusual case of fracture dislocation of the femur. JAMA 82: 1608
215. Haudidier P (1945) Contribution a l'étude des luxations traumatiques bilatérales de la hanche. Thesis, Nancy
216. Heim U, Pfeiffer K (1982) Small fragment set manual. Springer, Berlin Heidelberg New York
217. Heinzelmann P, Nelson C (1976) Recurrent traumatic dislocation of the hip. J Bone Joint Surg [Am] 58: 895-896
218. Helal B, Skevis X (1967) Unrecognised dislocation of the hip in fractures of the femoral shaft. J Bone Joint Surg [Br] 49: 293-300
219. Helferich (1893) Ueber die blutige Reposition von Luxationen. Dtsch Med Wochenschr 32: 761-763
220. Hennicke W (1973) Ein Beitrag zur traumatischen Hüftverrenkung im Kindesalter. Beitr Orthop 20: 641-644
221. Henry A, Bayumi M (1934) Fracture of the femur with luxation of the ipsilateral hip. Br J Surg 22: 204-230

222. Hensley C, Schofield G (1969) Recurrent dislocation of the hip. J Bone Joint Surg [Am] 51: 573-577
223. Hidalgos A: personal communication
224. Hidalgos A: personal communication
225. Higgins T (1920) Case of subluxation of right hip-joint, following trauma. Proc R Soc Med 21: 62-63
226. Hipp E (1969) Spätfolgen nach Hüftverletzungen im Kindesalter. Z Orthop 106: 609-622
227. Hofliger (1900) Die operative Behandlung irreponibler traumatischer Hüftgelenksluxationen. Dissertation, Bern
228. Hohmann D (1964) Rezidivierende traumatische Hüftluxation beim Kind nach fehlerhafter Gipsfixation. Monatsschr Unfallheilkd 67: 352-355
229. Hollingdale J, Aicroth P (1981) Recurrent post-traumatic dislocation of the hip in children. J R Soc Med 74: 545-546
230. Hovelius L (1974) Traumatic dislocation of the hip in children. Acta Orthop Scand 45: 746-751
231. Howe W, Lacey T, Schwartz R (1950) A study of the gross anatomy of the arteries supplying the proximal portion of the femur and the acetabulum. J Bone Joint Surg [Am] 32: 856-866
232. Hulth A (1957) The vessel anatomy of the upper femur end with special regards to the mechanism of trauma. Acta Orthop Scand 27: 192-197
233. Hunter G (1969) Posterior dislocation and fracture-dislocation of the hip. J Bone Joint Surg [Br] 51: 38-44
234. Ingram A, Bachynski B (1953) Fractures of the hip in children. J Bone Joint Surg [Am] 35: 867, 887
235. Ingram A, Turner T (1954) Bilateral traumatic posterior dislocation of the hip complicated by bilateral fracture of the femoral shaft. J Bone Joint Surg [Am] 36: 1249-1255
236. Jaberg H, Ganz R (1983) Komplikationen bei traumatischer Hüftgelenksluxation bei Kindern. Ther Umsch 40: 956-959
237. Jacobs B (1978) Epidemiology of traumatic and nontraumatic osteonecrosis. Clin Orthop 130: 51-67
237a. Jacquemain B (1967) Die Bedeutung der geburtstraumatischen Epiphysenlösung am proximalen Femurende. Geburtshilfe Frauenheilkd 27: 690-695
238. Jalaguier (1903) Luxation traumatique de la hanche gauche chez un enfant de dix ans: réduction après vingt-deux jours. Bull Mem Soc Chir 29: 879-880
239. Jansen U, Pedersen S (1979) Traumatisk hofteluksation hos born. Ugeskr Laeger 141: 2672-2673
240. Jantzen P (1958) Die Verletzungen des Hüftgelenkes und ihre Behandlung unter besonderer Berücksichtigung der Spätfolgen. Z Orthop 90: 55-78
241. Jazayeri M (1978) Posterior fracture-dislocation of the hip joint with emphasis on the importance of hip tomography in their management. Orthop Rev 7: 59-64
242. Jensen H (1955) Traumatic dislocation of the hip joint in childhood with avascular necrosis of the femoral head. J Oslo City Hosp 5: 101-105
243. Jenny G: personal communication
244. Johner R, Ganz R (1977) Traumatische Verletzungen der kindlichen Hüfte. Ther Umsch 34: 305-313
245. Jonasch E (1958) Traumatische kindliche Hüftverrenkungen. Z Orthop 90: 357-359
246. Jonasch E (1962) Traumatische Hüftluxation beim Kind. Verh Dtsch Orthop Ges 50: 291-293
247. Jones S (1884) Traumatic dislocation of hip; useless lim; excision of head of femur; successful result. Lancet 2: 870
248. Judet R: quoted by Barcat J, Testas P (Reference 19)
249. Judet R, Judet J, Letournel E (1964) Fractures of the acetabulum; classification and surgical approaches for open reduction. J Bone Joint Surg [Am] 46: 1615-1646
250. Jungbluth K, Kratzert R (1968) Spätergebnisse schwerer Hüftgelenksverletzungen. Arch Klin Chir 320: 8-25
251. Kalamchi A, MacEwen G (1980) Avascular necrosis following treatment of congenital dislocation of the hip. J Bone Joint Surg [Am] 62: 876-888
252. Kammerer F (1889) On the complication of dislocation with fracture of the femur, with a case. NY Med J 49: 175-180
253. Kanan S, Giordano J, Nunes R, Peixinho M: personal communication

254. Karehneke M (1907) Kasuistischer Beitrag zu Oberschenkelluxationen. Münch Med Wochenschr 35: 1738
255. Kaufmann: quoted by Hofliger (Reference 227)
256. Kenwright J (1977) Dislocation of the hip and acetabular fractues. In: Muckle D (ed) Femoral neck fractures and hip joint injuries. Chapman and Hall, London
257. Kirmisson: quoted by Piollet P (1901) Traitement sanglant des luxations traumatiques anciennes de la hanche. Thesis, Lyon
258. Klasen H (1979) Traumatic dislocation of the hip in children. Reconstr Surg Traumatol 17: 119-129
259. Klasen H, Binnendjk B (1984) Fracture of the neck of the femur associated with posterior dislocation of the hip. J Bone Joint Surg [Br] 66: 45-48
260. Klee F (1889) Ueber 32 traumatische Hüftgelenksluxationen. Beitr Klin Chir 4: 513-536
261. Klein A, Summer T, Volberg F, Orbon R (1982) Combined CT-arthrography in recurrent traumatic hip dislocation. AJR 138: 963-964
262. Kleinberg G (1939) Aseptic necrosis of the femoral head following traumatic dislocation. Arch Surg 39: 637-646
263. Klemm K: personal communication
264. Klems H (1972) Traumatische Hüftgelenksluxation im Kindesalter. Z Orthop 110: 579-582
265. Klisic P (1984) Perthes' disease. Int Orthop 8: 95-102
266. Kohn L (1973) Luxación traumática de cadera. Rev Ortop Traumatol Latinoam 18: 199-204
267. Koszla M (1963) Traumatic dislocation of the hip in children. Chir Narzadow Ruchu Ortop Pol 28: 565-568
268. Kroll H (1940) Sur la question de la luxation traumatique de la hanche chez les nouveau-nés. Thèse Erlangen
269. Kucerova K (1952) Traumatic hip dislocation in children. Acta Chir Orthop Traumatol Cech 19: 209-212
270. Kummer E (1891) Y a-t-il allongement ou raccourcissement du la jambe dans la luxation obturatrice régulière de la hanche. Rev Orthop 3: 133-136
271. Kuner E (1975) Die Indikationen zur Osteosynthese beim kindlichen Knochenbruch. Chirurg 46: 164-169
272. Kuster: quoted by Volkmann R (Reference 504)
273. Labaziewicz L (1976) Inveterate traumatic dislocation of the hip with necrosis of the femoral head in a child. Chir Narzadow Ruchu Ortop Pol 41: 5-7
274. Lagrange J, Dunoyer J (1962) La vascularisation de la tête fémorale de l'enfant. Rev Chir Orthop 48: 123-137
275. Lam S (1971) Fractures of the neck of the femur in children. J Bone Joint Surg [Am] 53: 1165-1177
276. Lane A: quoted by Gayet G (1902) De la réposition sanglante de la tête fémorale dans les luxations irréductibles de la hanche. Rev Chir 26: 280-292
277. Laskowski M, Mazurkiewicz S (1973) Traumatic dislocation of the hip joint in children. Chir Narzadow Ruchu Ortop Pol 38: 23-26
278. Lauritzen J (1975) Legg-Calvé-Perthes disease: a comparative study. Acta Orthop Scand [Suppl] 159
279. Lavianos I: personal communication
280. Lawrence H (1877) Dislocation of the right femur into the obturator foramen in a child. Lancet 1: 461-462
281. Lehtonen R (1968) A study of traumatic dislocation of the hip joint and fractures of the acetabulum. Ann Chir Gynaecol Fenn 57 [Suppl 163]
282. Lemoine A (1957) Vascular changes after interference with the blood flow of the femoral head of the rabbit. J Bone Joint Surg [Br] 39: 763-777
283. Lesourd G (1969) Luxation traumatique de la hanche droite, avec décollement épiphysaire de la tête fémorale et fracture du sourcil cityloïdien postérieur chez un enfant de 15 ans. Rev Chir Orthop 55: 61-64
284. Letenneur J, Rogez J, Leveau J, Maulaz D (1984) Luxations traumatiques pures de la hanche. Luxations de hanche et fractures de tête fémorale. Encycl Méd Chir (Paris, France). Appareil locomoteur, 14077 A10, 12-1984
285. Lezama L (1950) Luxación traumática reciente de cadera. Rev Ortop Traumatol 20: 153-159

286. Liber J: quoted by Cartron P (Reference 75)
287. Liebenberg F, Dommisse G (1969) Recurrent post-traumatic dislocation of the hip. J Bone Joint Surg [Br] 51: 632-637
288. Lievre C (1959) Della lussazione traumatica dell'anca. Min Ortop 10: 317-324
289. Litton L, Workman C (1958) Traumatic anterior dislocation of the hip in children. J Bone Joint Surg [Am] 49: 1419-1422
290. Liuboshits N (1963) Traumatic dislocation of the hip in children associated with pelvic fractures. Vestn Khir: 91: 94-97
291. Liuboshits N, Nemsadze V (1964) Traumatic dislocation of both hips with unilateral fracture of a hip in a child of 13 years. Khirurgiia (Mosk) 40: 146-148
292. Liuboshits N, Nemsadze V, Aiabyev V (1964) Traumatic dislocations of the hip in children. Ortop Travmatol Protez 25: 9-13
293. Loray J (1955) Luxación traumática de cadera en la infancia. Bol Trab Soc Arg Ortop Traumatol, Sesión del 31 de Mayo de 1955
294. Lovell W: discussion, following Simmons R, Elder J (Reference 458)
295. Lugger L (1974) Traumatische Hüftverrenkung und gleichseitiger Oberschenkelhalsbruch im Kindesalter. Zentralbl Chir 99: 340-342
295a. Lutter L (1973) Post-traumatic hip redislocation. J Bone Joint Surg [Am] 55: 391-394
296. Lyddon D, Hartman J (1971) Traumatic dislocation of the hip with ipsilateral femoral fracture. J Bone Joint Surg [Am] 53: 1012-1016
297. Macewen: quoted by Giraud D (Reference 184)
298. Macfarlane I, King D (1976) Traumatic dislocation of the hip joint in children. Aust NZ J Surg 46: 227-231
299. Mackay G: discussion, following Ghormley R, Sullivan R (Reference 181)
300. Maffei F (1922) Contributo allo stuido della lussazione traumatica dell'anca nell'infanzia. Chir Organi Mov 6: 604-624
301. Maia B (1936) Consideraçoes em torno das luxaçoes coxo-femurais traumaticas. Arq Bras Cir Ortop 4: 328-334
302. Maitrejean M (1924) Les luxations traumatiques de la hanche chez l'enfant. Thesis, Lyon
303. Malgaigne J (1855) Traité des fractures et des luxations. Bailliere, Paris
304. Malkawi H (1982) Traumatic anterior dislocation of the hip with fracture of the shaft of the ipsilateral femur in children. J Pediatr Orthop 2: 307-311
305. Markoe: quoted by Henry A, Bayumi M (Reference 221)
306. Martel F (1920) La luxation traumatique de la hanche chez l'enfant. Thesis, Nancy
307. Masliah R (1969) Tratamiento de las fracturas por el método de compresión. VII Congreso Argentino de Ortopedia y Traumatología, pp 131-135
308. Masliah R: personal communication
309. Mason M (1954) Traumatic dislocation of the hip in childhood. J Bone Joint Surg [Br] 36: 630-632
310. Mass D, Spiegel P, Laros G (1980) Dislocation of the hip with traumatic separation of the capital femoral epiphysis: report of a case with successful outcome. Clin Orthop 146: 184-187
311. Masse P, Florent J (1964) Une luxation récidivante de la hanche chez une fille de 6 ans. Rev Chir Orthop 50: 705-708
312. Matsubara T, Miyao M (1969) On avascular necrosis of the femoral head following traumatic hip dislocation. Orthop Surg 20: 892-899
313. Mau C (1953) Hüftluxation und Femurfraktur. Monatsschr Unfallheilkd 56: 225-230
314. Mauck H, Anderson R (1935) Infracotyloid dislocation of the hip. J Bone Joint Surg 17: 1011-1013
315. M'Bamali E (1975) Unusual traumatic anterior dislocation of the hip. Injury 6: 220-224
316. McDougall A (1961) Fractures of the neck of the femur in childhood. J Bone Joint Surg [Br] 43: 16-28
317. Meller Y, Tennenbaum Y, Torok G (1982) Subcapital fracture of neck of femur with complete posterior dislocation of the hip. J Trauma 22: 327-329
318. Meng C (1934) Traumatic dislocation of the hip in childhood. Clin Med J [Engl] 48: 736-737
319. Meyers M, Talfer N, Moore T (1977) Determination of the vascularity of the femoral head with technetium 99-m sulphur-colloid. Diagnostic and prognostic significance. J Bone Joint Surg [Am] 59: 658-665

320. Michel L (1938) Sur les luxations traumatiques de la hanche chez l'enfant. Rev Med Franc 19: 549-554
321. Michelmore G (1889) A case of old unreduced dislocation of hip. Lancet 2: 1224
322. Miglietta P (1969) Un caso di lussazione traumatica dell'anca in una bambina de 23 mesi. Chir Organi Mov 24: 383-389
323. Mikulicz: quoted by Drehmann G (Reference 129)
324. Milazzo S, Fiandaca C (1967) Sulle lussazioni traumatiche coxo-femorali della prima infanzia. Atti SOTIMI 15: 15-19
325. Moll J (1973) Fractures and dislocations of the hip joint. In: Tronzo R (ed) Surgery of the hip joint. Lea and Febiger, Philadelphia
326. Morton K (1959) Traumatic dislocation of the hip in children. Br J Surg 47: 233-237
327. Mossakowska B (1964) Traumatic dislocation of the hip in a 2-year-old child. Chir Narzadow Ruchu Ortop Pol 29: 53-55
328. Motta C (1965) Probleme der veralteten traumatischen Hüftverrenkungen. Z Orthop 100: 133-153
329. Mouchet A, Seguinot (1910) Deux cas de luxations traumatiques de la hanche chez l'enfant. Rev Orthop 3: 553-558
330. Mouczy: quoted by Giraud D (Reference 184)
331. Muller M (1974) Schenkelhalsfraktur beim Kind. Orthop Praxis 2: 65-67
332. Muller M, Ganz R (1974) Luxationen und Frakturen der unteren Gliedmaßen und Becken. In: Rehn J (ed) Unfallverletzungen bei Kindern. Springer, Berlin Heidelberg New York
333. Muller M, Allgower M, Schneider R, Willenegger H (1979) Manual of internal fixation. Springer, Berlin Heidelberg New Yor
334. Murphy D (1923) Traumatic luxation of the hip in childhood. JAMA 80: 549
335. Mutschler H (1939) Sekundäre Oberschenkelkopfnekrose nach traumatischer Ausrenkung des Hüftgelenkes bei einem 14 Jährigen. Münch Med Wochenschr 86: 258-260
336. Nathan W (1928) Geburtstrauma und Hüftgelenksverrenkung. Z Orthop 49: 383-387
337. Naeraa A (1938) On secondary epiphyseal necrosis after collum femoris fracture in young persons. Acta Chir Scand 80: 238-250
338. Nelson C (1970) Traumatic recurrent dislocation of the hip. J Bone Joint Surg [Am] 52: 128-130
339. Nerubay J (1976) Traumatic anterior dislocation of hip joint with vascular damage. Clin Orthop 116: 129-132
340. Newman J (1973) Posterior dislocation of the hip with ipsilateral subcapital fracture of the neck of the femur, treated conservatively: a case report. Injury 5: 329-331
341. Nicolaysen K (1931) Malum coxae Calvé-Legg-Perthes' potagenese, belyst ved et enkelt tilfelle. Norsk Mag Laegevidensk 92: 985-989
342. Niloff P, Petrie J (1950) Traumatic anterior dislocation of the hip. Can Med Assoc J 62: 574-576
343. Nielsen B (1938) Om Calve-Perthes sygdom after fractura col femoris hos unge og dens betydnig forstaaelsen af aseptiiske epifysenekroser patogenese. Hospitals 81: 773-782
344. Niradi L et al (1980) Surgical treatment of traumatic hip dislocation in childhood. Ortop Travmatol Protez 41: 61-62
345. Nixon J (1976) Late open reduction of traumatic dislocation of the hip. J Bone Joint Surg [Br] 58: 41-43
346. Obel W, Debowska-Wojcik D (1976) Traumatic hip luxation in children in the light of clinical observations. Pediatr Pol 51: 689-694
347. Oelrich H, Machan F (1972) Doppelseitige und kindliche traumatische Hüftluxationen, seltene Formen der Hüftluxation. Z Ärztl Fortbild (Jena) 66: 807-811
348. Offierski C (1981) Traumatic dislocation of the hip in children. J Bone Joint Surg [Br] 63: 194-197
349. Ogden J (1974) Changing patterns of proximal femoral vascularity. J Bone Joint Surg [Am] 56: 941-950
350. Ogden J (1981) Hip development and vascularity: relationship to chondro-osseous trauma in the growing child. In: Salvatti EA (ed) The hip. Mosby, St. Louis
351. Ogden J (1982) Skeletal injury in the child. Lea and Febiger, Philadelphia
352. Ogden J, Lee K, Rudicel S, Pelker R (1984) Proximal femoral epiphyseolysis in the neonate. J Pediatr Orthop 4: 285-292

353. Ollier L (1891) Traité des resections. Masson, Paris
354. Oni O, Orhewere F, Keswani H (1984) The treatment of old unreduced traumatic dislocations of the hip. Injury 15: 219-223
355. Oprandi C, Sette F (1962) La lussazione traumatica dell'anca con frattura del ciglio cotiloideo. Arch Ortop 75: 874-892
356. Oprandi C (1969) Contributo allo studio della lussazione traumatica dell'anca nell'infanzia. Clin Ortop 21: 86-94
357. Ormerod (1847) Clinical collections and observations in surgery made during an attendance on the surgical practice of St. Bartholomew's Hospital. Am J Med Sci 4: 182
358. Osborne G, Cotterill P (1966) Recurrent dislocation of the elbow. J Bone Joint Surg [Br] 48: 340-346
359. Ostapowicz G (1968) Traumatische Hüftgelenksluxation bei einem 4jährigen Knaben. Monatsschr Unfallheilkd 71: 207-213
360. Ottolenghi C: discussion, following Ayerza I, González L, Silvetti R: Luxación traumática inveterada de la cadera. Bol Trab Soc Arg Ortop Traumatol, Sesión del 25 de Julio de 1950
361. Pagano G, Petazzi I, Mosoni P (1976) La lussazione traumatica dell'anca nel bambino. Min Ortop 27: 133-141
362. Paltrinieri M (1938) Epifisiti tardive conseguenti a lussazioni traumatiche dell'anca. Boll Soc Med (Bologna) 110: 124-128
363. Pannike A (1979) Pathophysiologie und Systematik der Ligamentarien Beckenverletzungen und der traumatischen Hüftverrenkungen. Hefte Unfallheilkd 140: 205-220
364. Paterson I (1957) The torn acetabular labrum. A block to reduction of a dislocated hip. J Bone Joint Surg [Br] 39: 306-309
365. Paus B (1951) Traumatic dislocations of the hip. Acta Orthop Scand 21: 99-112
366. Pearson D, Mann R (1973) Traumatic hip dislocation in children. Clin Orthop 92: 189-194
367. Peiliski M, Busczynski A (1971) Dislocations of the hip joint with fracture of the femoral shaft. Chir Narzadow Ruchu Ortop Pol 36: 19-24
368. Peltokallio P, Kurkipaa M (1959) Fractures of the femoral neck in children. Ann Chir Gynaecol Fenn 48: 152-163
369. Pennsylvania Orthopedic Society (1960) Traumatic dislocation of the hip joint in children. J Bone Joint Surg [Am] 42: 705-710
370. Pennsylvania Orthopaedic Society (1968) Traumatic dislocation of the hip joint in children. Final report. J Bone Joint Surg [Am] 50: 79-88
371. Perrando I (1900) Casistica di chirurgia ortopedica: riposizione cruenta di lussazione inveterata del femore. Arch Ortop 17: 7-11
372. Perruelo N: discussion, following Loray J (Reference 293)
373. Perry B (1966) Traumatic dislocation of the hip in the child. Am Surg 32: 419-420
374. Peschties (1908) Ueber spontane und traumatische Luxationen des Hüftgelenkes im Kindesalter. Dissertation, Königsberg
375. Peterson L (1950) Dislocation of the hip associated with fracture of the neck of the femur. J Bone Joint Surg [Am] 37: 274-279
376. Petrini A, Grassi G (1983) Long term results in traumatic dislocation of the hip in children. Ital J Orthop Traumatol 9: 225-230
377. Pfab B (1938) Endausgänge von traumatischen Hüftgelenksverrenkungen. Arch Orthop Unfall-Chir 39: 135-143
378. Pfeiffer (1887) A case of double dislocation of the hips. Boston Med Surg J 67: 103
379. Pforringer W, Rosemeyer B (1977) Schenkelhalsfrakturen im Kindesalter. Arch Orthop Unfall-Chir 88: 281-308
380. Phemister D (1934) Fractures of neck of femur, dislocation of hip and obscure vascular disturbances producing aseptic necrosis of head of femur. Surg Gynecol Obstet 59: 415-440
381. Picchio A (1956) Le lussazioni traumatiche dell'anca nell'infanzia. Clin Ortop 8: 419-426
382. Pidhorz L, Mouterde P (1974) Luxations traumatiques pures de la hanche. Encycl Méd Chir (Paris, France). Appareil Locomoteur, 14901 B10, 3-1974
383. Pietrafesa C, Hoffman J (1983) Traumatic dislocation of the hip. JAMA 249: 3342-3346
384. Pietrzikowski: quoted by Doelle O (Reference 124)
385. Piggot J (1961) Traumatic dislocation of the hip in childhood. J Bone Joint Surg [Br] 43: 38-42

386. Pipkin G (1957) Treatment of grade IV fracture-dislocation of the hip. J Bone Joint Surg [Am] 39: 1027-1042
387. Piqué J, Ottolenghi E (1937) Luxación ilíaca traumática de la cadera. Rev Asoc Méd Hosp Durand 4: 70-74
388. Pirotto J (1968) Fractura de pared posterior de cotilo con luxación de cadera y parálisis ciática. In: Lesiones traumáticas de pelvis. Oficina del Libro-AEM, Montevideo
389. Pizio Z (1971) Traumatic anterior luxation of the hip joint in children. Wiad Lek 24: 149-153
390. Pizio Z (1971) Long-term results of hip arthroplasty performed for a primary undiagnosed traumatic hip dislocation with simultaneous fracture of the shaft of the femur. Chir Narzadow Ruchu Ortop Pol 36: 317-321
391. Pizziolo I (1964) Un eccezionale caso di lussazione d'anca intra-partum. Chir Organi Mov 19: 464-469
392. Platt H, von Mengershausen H (1916) Traumatic dislocation of the hip-joint in a child. Lancet 1: 80
393. Post: quoted by Henry A, Bayumi M (Reference 221)
394. Pouliquen E (1956) Luxation traumatique de la hanche au cours de l'accouchement par siège. Ouest Med 7: 99-101
395. Pous J, Dimeglio A (1978) La hanche en croissance. Bailliere, Paris
396. Pouzet F (1932) Sur la fragmentation de l'épiphyse fémorale de l'enfant. Arch Franco-Belges Chir 33: 535-541
397. Powdrell J (1868) Case of dislocation of the hip-joint in a child six months old. Lancet 1: 617
398. Prat D, Roca B (1973) Luxación traumática de cadera en niños. An Hosp S Cruz y S Pablo 17: 249-258
399. Princeteau A (1921) Considérations sur un cas de luxation traumatique ovalaire de la hanche chez un enfant. Thesis, Bordeaux
400. Proctor H (1974) Dislocations of the hip joint (excluding "central" dislocation) and their complications. Injury 5: 1-12
401. Psathakis N (1964) Die übersehene Hüftluxation bei multiplen Verletzungen. Monatsschr Unfallheilkd 67: 224-229
402. Quist-Hanssen S (1945) Caput necrosis after traumatic dislocation of the hip joint in a 4-year-old boy, and control examinations of 8 cases of luxatio coxae traumatica. Acta Chir Scand 92: 393-402
403. Quist-Hanssen S (1947) Supplement to: Caput necrosis after traumatic dislocation of the hip joint in a 4-year-old boy, and control examinations of 8 cases of luxatio coxae traumatica. Acta Chir Scand 95: 344-346
404. Ralis Z, McKibbin B (1973) Changes in shape of the human hip joint during its development and their relation to its stability. J Bone Joint Surg [Br] 55: 780-785
405. Rampoldi A, Scoccianti P (1958) Lussazione traumatica d'anca nell'infanzia tratatta con artroplastica con capsula acrilica. Ortop Traumatol App Mot 26: 187-198
406. Rang M (1974) Children's fractures. Lippincott, Philadelphia
407. Rao J, Read R (1975) Luxatio erecta of the hip. Clin Orthop 110: 137-138
408. Ratliff A (1962) Fractures of the neck of the femur in children. J Bone Joint Surg [Br] 44: 528-542
409. Ravaglia M, Zorzi C (1955) Fratture dell collo e della diafisi femorale associate. Chir Organi Mov 41: 276-289
409a. Rees D, Thompson S (1984) Traumatic dislocation of the hip in mini rugby. Br Med J 289: 19-20
410. Rehbein M (1922) Zur Ätiologie der Perthesschen Krankheit, zugleich ein Beitrag zur traumatischen Hüftgelenksluxation im Kindesalter. Dtsch Z Chir 174: 416-423
410a. Reigstad A (1980) Traumatic dislocation of the hip. J Trauma 20: 603-606
411. Rendu A, Maitrejean M (1924) Les luxations traumatiques de la hanche chez l'enfant. Rev Orthop 11: 497-515
412. Ricci F, De Angelis Ricciotti F (1963) Sulla lussazione traumatica dell'anca nell'infanzia. Atti SOTIMI 8: 235-245
413. Rigault P, Hannouche D, Judet J (1968) Luxations traumatiques de la hanche et fractures du cotyle chez l'enfant. Rev Chir Orthop 54: 361-382
414. Riedel: quoted by Henry A, Bayumi M (Reference 221)

415. Rinke W, Protze J (1976) Offene traumatische Hüftgelenksluxation und gleichseitige Oberschenkelschaftfraktur im Kindesalter. Zentralbl Chir 101: 177-179
416. Rischbieth H (1914) Traumatic dislocation of the hip-joint occurring in a boy 10 years old. Lancet 1: 1111
417. Ritchey S, Schonholtz G, Thompson M (1958) The dashboard femoral fracture. J Bone Joint Surg [Am] 40: 1347-1358
418. Ritter G, Hollwarth M, Hausbrandt D, Linhart W (1984) Die traumatische Hüftluxation im Kindesalter. Unfallheilkunde 87: 24-26
419. Rivington W (1878) Some cases of dislocations of the hip and shoulder joints. Lancet 2: 321-322
420. Robertson R, Peterson H (1974) Traumatic dislocation of hip in children: review of Mayo Clinic series. In: Harris WH (ed) The hip. Mosby, St. Louis
421. Rocher H, Rocher C, Cuzard M (1937) Luxation traumatique de la hanche chez l'enfant. Bordeaux Chir 8: 255-261
422. Roeder L, De Lee J (1980) Femoral head fractures associated with posterior hip dislocations. Clin Orthop 147: 121-130
423. Roederer C (1912) La luxation traumatique de la hanche chez l'enfant. Paris Med 7: 604-606
424. Roello G (1916) Contributo allo studio della lussazione traumatica dell'anca nell'infanzia. Clin Chir 24: 1480-1502
425. Roello G (1922) Sulla lussazione traumatica dell'anca nell'infanzia. Chir Organi Mov 6: 119-124
426. Rogala P, Labaziewicz L (1977) An old traumatic hip dislocation associated with fracture of the femoral diaphysis in a child, complicated by avascular necrosis of the femoral head. Chir Narzadow Ruchu Ortop Pol 42: 265-267
427. Rosa D (1983) Considerazioni su di un raro caso di distacco-frattura-lussazione del nucleo cefalico femorale. Chir Organi Mov 68: 741-746
428. Rosemberg (1897) Zur operativen Behandlung der irreponiblen traumatischen Hüftgelenksluxationen. Dissertation, Göttingen
429. Roux (1913) Luxation de la hanche: résultats éloignés. Rev Med Suisse Romande 33: 1-35
430. Rowe C (1974) Dislocation of the hip and fractures of the acetabulum. In: Cave E, Burke J, Boyd R (eds) Trauma management. Year Book Medical, Chicago
431. Ruffoni R (1962) Su un raro caso di lussazione traumatica bilaterale d'anca associato a distacco epifisario prossimale del femore sinistro. Arch Ortop 75: 325-333
432. Ruiz Moreno I: discussion, following Loray J (Reference 293)
433. Russe O: quoted by Sarungi P (Reference 438)
434. Salina-Borello G, Zarcone P (1975) La lussazione traumatica dell'anca nell'infanzia. Min Ortop 26: 212-214
435. Sandor L, Nyirady L, Jokai I (1979) Traumatische Hüftluxation im Kindesalter - Einkrempelung der Pfannenkante als Repositionshindernis. Beitr Orthop Traumatol 26: 32-37
436. Sanguinetti C (1967) Le fratture dell collo del femore nel bambino. Boll Mem Soc Tosco-Umbra di Chirurgica 28: 455-465
437. Sankarankutty M (1967) Traumatic inferior dislocation of the hip (luxatio erecta) in a child. J Bone Joint Surg [Br] 49: 145
438. Sarungi P (1974) Traumatic posterior dislocation of the hip in a child. East Afr Med J 51: 364-369
439. Sauser D, Billimoria P, Rouse G, Mudge K (1980) CT evaluation of hip trauma. AJR 135: 269-274
440. Schiele E (1947) Traumatische Hüftgelenksluxation mit Femurkopfepiphysenlösung und ihre Behandlung durch Kopfresektion und Fascientransplantation. Chirurg 17: 703-708
441. Schlonsky J, Miller P (1973) Traumatic hip dislocation in children. J Bone Joint Surg [Am] 55: 1057-1063
442. Schoenecker P, Manske P, Sertl G (1978) Traumatic hip dislocation with ipsilateral femoral shaft fractures. Clin Orthop 130: 233-238
443. Scholder C (1955) Le traitement orthopédique des dystrophies de l'extrémité supérieure du fémur. Rev Orthop 41: 73-91
444. Scholder-Dumur C (1959) Nécrose de la tête fémorale à la suite de luxation traumatique de la hanche chez l'enfant. Rev Chir Orthop 45: 504-505

445. Schomann: quoted by Streissler E (Reference 474)
446. Schonbauer H (1961) Begleitverletzungen am Oberschenkel bei Hüftverrenkungen. Klin Med 16: 39-41
447. Schwartz D, Haller J (1974) Open anterior hip dislocation with femoral vessel transection in a child. J Trauma 14: 1054-1059
448. Scialpi G, Bonaventura R (1967) Sulla lussazione traumatica dell'anca nell'infanzia. Atti SOTIMI 16: 1-7
449. Scott J, Thomas F (1974) Delayed presentation of post-traumatic posterior dislocation of the hip with acetabular rim fracture. Injury 5: 325-326
450. Seddon H (1972) Surgical disorders of the peripheral nerves. Churchill Livingstone, Edinburgh
451. Sedillot: quoted by Giraud D (Reference 184)
452. Seewald R (1960) Traumatische Hüftgelenksluxationen bei Kindern und Jugendlichen. Arch Orthop Unfall-Chir 51: 635-638
453. Seiderer: quoted by Maffei F (Reference 300)
454. Seringe R, Lance D (1983) Fractures de la diaphyse fémorale chez l'enfant. Encyl Méd Chir, Paris, Appareil locomoteur, 14078 B10, 2-1983
455. Shim S (1979) Circulatory and vascular changes in the hip following traumatic hip dislocation. Clin Orthop 140: 255-261
456. Shina D, Kumar M (1983) Traumatic dislocation of hip joint in children in Chotanagpur. J Indian Med Assoc 80: 23-25
457. Siffert R (1981) Deformities caused by injuries to the growing hip. In: Salvatti EA (ed) The hip. Mosby, St. Louis
458. Simmons R, Elder J (1972) Recurrent posttraumatic dislocation of the hip in children. South Med J 65: 1463-1466
459. Silveri A, Castiglioni N (1973) Tratamiento de la luxación congénita de la cadera. Cir Urug 43 [Suppl 5]
460. Slatis P, Latvala A (1974) Irreducible traumatic posterior dislocation of the hip. Injury 5: 188-193
461. Slullitel J: discussion, following Loray J (Reference 293)
462. Smith K (1887) A case of dislocation of the hip in a child aged five. Lancet 1: 417
463. Smith M: personal communication
464. Snook G, Chrisman O (1965) Interposition of the joint capsule in traumatic posterior dislocation of the hip. J Trauma 5: 358-361
465. Soares L: personal communication
466. Sommerville E (1982) Displacement of the hip in childhood. Springer, Berlin Heidelberg New York
467. Speed K (1942) A text-book of fractures and dislocations. Lea and Febiger, Philadelphia
468. Spencer (1895) Traumatic hip dislocation in a child. Br Med J 1: 366
469. Spissak L, Kirnak J, Stojkovic J (1969) Traumatic dislocation of the hip in children. Bratisl Lek Listy 52: 464-468
470. Steinke: quoted by Maffei F (Reference 300)
471. Sterling R, Meade T (1982) Traumatic dislocation of the hip in children. Orthop Trans 6: 94
472. Sternberg H (1933) Zur Kenntnis der Hüftgelenksverletzungen im Kindesalter. Arch Orthop Unfall-Chir 33: 250-255
473. Stewart M, Milford L (1954) Fracture-dislocation of the hip. J Bone Joint Surg [Am] 36: 315-334
474. Streissler E (1908) Ueber die operative Behandlung irreponibler vorderer Hüftluxationen. Beitr Klin Chir 58: 571-605
475. Stringa G (1955) Un caso di lussazione d'anca intra-partum. Chir Organi Mov 41: 448-452
476. Suero C, Queirolo J, Ceballos R (1973) Enfermedad de Perthes. Cir Urug 43 [Suppl 5]
477. Suero C, Schimchak M (1978) Anatomía macroscópica de la extremidad superior del fémur en el niño. Acta Ortop Latinoam 5: 41-48
478. Sullivan C, Bickel W, Lipscomb P (1955) Recurrent dislocation of the hip. J Bone Joint Surg [Am] 37: 1266-1270
479. Sundt H (1920) Malum coxae Calvé-Legg-Perthes. Z Chir 47: 538-542
480. Tailhefer A: A propos de la communication de Barcat J, Testas P (Reference 19)

481. Tile M (1980) Fractures of the acetabulum. Orthop Clin North Am 11: 481-506
482. Titze A (1960) Eine traumatische Hüftgelenksverrenkung beim Kind mit Repositionshindernis. Arch Orthop Unfall-Chir 52: 259-264
483. Titze A (1961) Untere Gliedmaßen. In: Ehalt W (ed) Verletzungen bei Kindern und Jugendlichen. Ferdinand Enke, Stuttgart
484. Townsend R, Edwards G, Bazant F (1969) Post-traumatic recurrent dislocation of the hip. J Bone Joint Surg [Br] 51: 194
485. Traversa C, Vázquez G, Ortolan E, Barrera E (1978) Lesión nerviosa en los traumatismos graves de la cadera. Acta Ortop Latinoam 5: 21-34
486. Trillat A, Ringot A (1951) Erreure d'interpretation radiographique dans les fractures du cotyle avec luxation de la tête fémorale. Lyon Chir 46: 472-474
487. Trojan E (1954) La miosite ossificante da lussazioni e fratture-lussazioni traumatiche d'anca. Chir Organi Mov 40: 129-134
488. Trojan E (1959) Luxation et fractures-luxations traumatiques de la hanche à l'exception des fractures-luxations avec enfoncement du cotyle. Rev Chir Orthop 45: 469-486
489. Tronzo R (1961) Traumatic dislocation of the hip in a child. A problem in anesthetic management. JAMA 176: 526-527
489a. Tronzo R (1984) Fractures of the femoral in children. In: Tronzo R (ed) Surgery of the hip. Springer, Berlin Heidelberg New York
490. Truchet: quoted by Martel F (Reference 306)
491. Trueta J (1957) The normal vascular anatomy of the human femoral head during growth. J Bone Joint Surg [Br] 39: 358-394
492. Trueta J (1975) La estructura del cuerpo humano. Estudio sobre su desarrollo y decadencia. Labor, Barcelona
493. Tuchten: quoted by Maffei F (Reference 300)
494. Ulloa I (1962) Traumatische Hüftgelenksverrenkung bei Kindern. Verh Dtsch Orthop Ges 50: 294-308
495. Upadhyay S, Moulton A (1981) The long-term results of traumatic posterior dislocation of the hip. J Bone Joint Surg [Br] 63: 548-551
496. Urist M (1947) Injuries to the hip joint. Am J Surg 74: 586-589
497. Vaeza E, Grille V (1973) Fracturas del cotilo. Cir Urug 43 [Suppl 5]
498. Vanni E, Franceschi A (1964) Lussazioni traumatiche e lussazioni-fratture della coxo-femorale con particolare riguardo agli esiti. Min Ortop 15: 51-62
499. Vécsei V (1975) Zur operativen Versorgung der Hüftverrenkungsbrüche. Arch Orthop Unfall-Chir 82: 107-121
500. Vécsei V: personal communication
501. Vena P, Pillitteri V (1970) La lussazione traumatica dell'anca nell'infanzia. Clin Ortop 22: 37-40
502. Verbrugge J (1955) Luxation postérieure de la hanche compliquée d'une fracture de la tête et de la diaphyse fémorales. Acta Orthop Belg 21: 357-364
503. Vetu P (1835) Considérations sur le traitement de la luxation du fémur en bas et en dédans sur le trou obturateur, suivies d'une observation de réduction par un procédé particulier. Thesis, Paris
504. Volkmann R (1893) Ueber die blutige Reposition veralteter traumatischer Hüftgelenksluxationen. Dtsch Z Chir 37: 373-390
505. Vrbecky J (1962) Traumatic dislocation of the hip joint in a new-born child. Acta Chir Orthop Traumatol Cech 29: 189-192
506. Wadsworth T (1961) Traumatic dislocation of the hip with fracture of the shaft of the ipsilateral femur. J Bone Joint Surg [Br] 43: 47-49
507. Warren J: quoted by Hamilton F (Reference 210)
508. Watkins J (1923) Obturator dislocation. J Bone Joint Surg 21: 243-259
509. Waters R (1972) Occult trauma in head injured victims of motor vehicle accidents. In: Orthopaedic seminars. Rancho Los Amigos Hospital, CA
510. Watson-Jones R (1960) Fractures and joint injuries. Livingstone, Edinburgh
511. Weber B, Brunner C, Freuler F (1980) Treatment of fractures in children and adolescents. Springer, Berlin Heidelberg New York
512. Weigand H, Schweikert C (1979) Spätergebnisse nach reinen traumatischen Hüftluxationen im Kindes- und Erwachsenenalter. Hefte Unfallheilkd 140: 239-248

513. Weil: quoted by Choyce C (Reference 105)
514. Werkman D (1980) The transepiphyseal fracture of the femoral neck. Injury 12: 50-52
515. Williams (1878) Probable ischiatic dislocation reduced after five months in a boy of eight years. Lancet 1: 86
516. Williams: quoted by Giraud D (Reference 184)
517. Wilson J (1976) Watson-Jones fractures and joint injuries. Livingstone, Edinburgh
518. Wilson D (1924) Displacement of upper epiphysis of femur treated by open reduction. JAMA 83: 1749-1756
519. Wilson D (1966) Traumatic dislocation of the hip in children: a report of four cases. J Trauma 6: 739-743
520. Wiltberger B, Mitchell C, Hedrick D (1948) Fracture of the femoral shaft complicated by hip dislocation. J Bone Joint Surg [Am] 30: 225-228
521. Wolcott W (1943) The evolution of the circulation in the developing femoral head and neck. Surg Gynecol Obstet 77: 61-69
522. Wood J (1852) Case of luxation of both hip-joints. NY Med Times 2: 33-34
523. Zarotti F (1951) Esiti di lussazione traumatica recente dell'anca. Min Ortop 2: 153-156
524. Zarotti F, Albertini B (1953) Trattamento ed esiti della lussazione traumatica inveterata dell'anca. Chir Organi Mov 39: 292-307

Subject Index

MIX
Papier aus verantwortungsvollen Quellen
Paper from responsible sources
FSC® C105338

If you have any concerns about our products,
you can contact us on
ProductSafety@springernature.com

In case Publisher is established outside the EU,
the EU authorized representative is:
Springer Nature Customer Service Center GmbH
Europaplatz 3, 69115 Heidelberg, Germany

Printed by Libri Plureos GmbH
in Hamburg, Germany